W9-BQK-517

It Shouldn't Be This Way

It Shouldn't Be This Way

The Failure of Long-Term Care

Robert L. Kane, M. D.
and
Joan C. West

VANDERBILT UNIVERSITY PRESS
Nashville

© 2005 Vanderbilt University Press
All rights reserved
First Edition 2005
10 09 08 07 06   2 3 4 5 6

Printed on acid-free paper
Manufactured in the United States of America
Design by Gary Gore

Library of Congress Cataloging-in-Publication Data
Kane, Robert L., 1940–
It shouldn't be this way : the failure of long-term care /
Robert L. Kane and Joan C. West.—1st ed. p. ; cm.
Includes bibliographical references and index.
ISBN 0-8265-1487-1 (cloth : alk. paper)
ISBN 0-8265-1488-X (pbk. : alk. paper)
    1. Older people—Long-term care—United States—Case
studies. 2. Kane, Ruth, d. 2002. 3. Kane, Robert L., 1940–
4. West, Joan C., 1945- 5. Caregivers—United States Biography.
6. Frail elderly—United States—Biography. 7. Long-term care
facilities—United States—Case studies. 8. Frail elderly—Care—
United States—Case studies. 9. Frail elderly—United States—
Family relationships—Case studies.
    [DNLM: 1. Long-Term Care—psychology—Personal Narratives.
2. Family—psychology—Personal Narratives.
3. Homes for the Aged—organization & administration—Personal
Narratives. 4. Nursing Homes—organization & administration—
Personal Narratives. WT 31 K156i 2005]
I. West, Joan C., 1945–   II. Title.
RA997.K355 2005
362.61'0973—dc22   2004028921

Contents

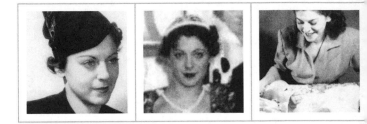

From left to right: As a hat model
before her marriage, circa 1932;
wedding photo, 1936; looking
at Joan as a baby, 1945; on
a cruise with her husband, 1968;
visiting Robert, 1983; on a date,
1989; in assisted living, 2001.

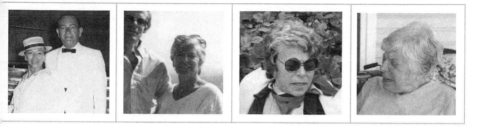

*We dedicate this book
to our mother, Ruth Kane,
who did not want her life to end
this way, in the hope that her
experiences will inspire others to
act. We hope, too, that her
grandchildren will not have
to share a similar fate.*

Introduction

The demand for long-term care is increasing steadily. It is the country's best-kept embarrassing secret. Almost every adult in this country will either enter a nursing home or have to deal with a parent or other relative who does. Demographic studies suggest that 40 percent of all adults in this country who live to age sixty-five will enter a nursing home before they die. Even more will use some other form of long-term care. Few people, however, are aware of this growing demand and few are prepared to deal with a system that is seriously flawed.

Some people believe that the key to dealing with long-term care is adequate preparation. Buying insurance and considering options for care should suffice. Alas, even these steps are not sufficient. You simply cannot rehearse the trials that long-term care subjects you to. That is why the system has to change. It is not enough to simply leave it up to each of us to be better prepared. Why should we gird up to battle a bad system?

Most people who confront this situation do so for the first time. Few people rehearse for this challenge. Few emerge unscarred. Despite all the theoretical discussions you might have had about what you would do, it is suddenly thrust upon you. Most of us face it with one parent, sometimes two; but the circumstances always seem unique and the challenges new. Even those of us who spend their careers studying the phenomenon are not really prepared for the reality of dealing with it firsthand.

Our mother, Ruth Kane, died in a nursing home on May 29, 2002. She was eighty-seven years old. Her death brought an end to a journey she had never wanted to make. Along the way she had experienced the very things she dreaded most. A woman who was vital and active three years earlier, who used to spend hours coordinating her wardrobe, had spent her last days wearing sweat suits and living in a barely furnished room with few of the possessions she had acquired over a lifetime. She had become disabled to the point where she was heavily dependent on others. She had lost her sense of dignity, to say nothing of the elegance she aspired to. In a sense she died some time earlier. The person we associated with our feisty, outspoken, independent mother had been replaced by a frail, demented old woman.

It was clear for several days that our mother was likely to die. She had had prior episodes of pulmonary illness and had recovered, but this one seemed worse. The attending physician was in regular contact with her son, Robert, also a physician, who lived in Minnesota. Her daughter, Joan, visited daily. Robert planned to come in a few days.

Early on the day our mother died, we felt that she was improving a little but that the end was likely in sight. Joan had a premonition. She actually visited our mother twice that day. Then she returned again when the nursing home physician called to say that her mother was dying. Joan and her husband rushed to our mother's bedside. She was still in the bed but so blue and cold. Joan kissed her and held her hand for a while. Her face was very peaceful. Joan felt quite numb. But it was finally over, and Joan experienced a mix of profound sadness and enormous relief. The staff members were kind, but it was the night group and Joan did not know them as well as she knew those who worked during the day. There was no sense of shared experience or shared loss.

Joan called her brother at once. Robert felt a sense of failure. He should have been there. He had chosen instead to visit his grandchildren in San Francisco, thinking that he still had a few days to make his last visit to his mother. He had seen her a few weeks earlier and though he had never really said good-bye, he had already done his grieving. And so to him, too, at the end, her death seemed like a relief from her having to live the life she feared the most.

Packing up our mother's few remaining possessions, we felt that her life should mean more than these fragments. Because her story is being repeated over and over again by many older people who face an uncertain and unwelcome experience in long-term care today, we decided to write this book. We want to share our experiences in caring for our mother with those who will face similar challenges and outline lessons that the care system and those who will depend on it need to heed to make the system more responsive to those whose lives it will dramatically alter.

Our story is certainly not unique, and that makes it worse. Many families face similar challenges but with far fewer resources from which to draw. Our intellectual and material resources make the story all the more tragic. We were two highly educated people negotiating a system that one of us made his life's work. Robert is a physician and gerontologist who has spent most of his professional career studying aging and its treatment. He holds an endowed chair in long-term care and aging at the University of Minnesota School of Public Health. His wife is a well-known gerontological social worker. They are both frequently away from their home in Minneapolis giving lectures or consulting. Joan, who lives and works in Long Island, holds a master's degree in elementary education and now trains future teachers. She was working full time teaching fourth grade students when our mother's episode of long-term care began.

Moreover, our mother had substantial financial resources. Though not wealthy by most standards, she had saved carefully and had amassed sizeable assets. These would prove enough to allow her to purchase care for many years. If we had many problems dealing with the myriad issues that surround terminal illness and long-term care, what must others face who are likely to be less well prepared?

For someone who smoked two packs of cigarettes a day until she was seventy, Ruth Kane was reasonably healthy into her eighties. Over the years, she weathered several serious threats to her health, and her reactions said a lot about how she wanted to deal with illness. When she was eighty-two, routine examinations uncovered a mass in her breast and an abnormal pap smear, which turned out to be a localized cancer. She adamantly refused treatment for either one, saying that she hated the thought of surgery and would probably die of something else long before they got her. She feared the pain that cancer might bring but not enough to do anything about it. She was especially concerned about the threat of mutilation from breast surgery, even resisting a lumpectomy. Despite our best efforts, she remained absolutely opposed to any further treatment. Subsequent events proved her right. Although she was very independent, she also had great respect for doctors and tended to acquiesce to their recommendations, except in the case of these two cancers.

Ruth was not wholly opposed to medical care, however. Many

years earlier she had been found to have a lymphoma in her groin and did agree to have it treated, even submitting to a course of chemotherapy in a hospital. Her aversion to pain and surgery could be overcome when it came to her physical appearance. She underwent a painful vein-stripping procedure to treat varicose veins. She had a lens implant for cataracts, which never healed well, and she suffered with vision problems for much of her older life.

Ruth's appearance was a major part of her identity. She loved to be admired. She had always been an attractive woman who put a lot of effort into maintaining her wardrobe and her appearance. When she was well beyond the age of Medicare, she reveled in the idea that even as she aged she was still regarded as an attractive woman. She rejected any threat to that image, including the need to wear low-heeled shoes to formal events. She regularly considered cosmetic surgery but never actually underwent any.

Becoming disabled was our mother's greatest fear. She repeated her fear regularly in many of our conversations and tried to exact promises from both of us that we would kill her before that could happen. Presumably she expected that Robert would have the knowledge and access to grant this boon. Discussions about the moral and legal difficulties of fulfilling her request did not dampen her enthusiasm and she never missed an opportunity to bring it up. Every encounter with someone gravely disabled led her to remark that she did not want to end up like that.

This story is thus a tragedy. Ruth's last three years were not the life she wanted. Despite the best efforts of two intelligent, informed, motivated, and well-connected children, one of whom is a prominent geriatric physician, the elder care health system could not adequately meet her needs. Ruth did have some moments when she seemed to feel genuine pleasure, and the people involved in the long-term care system often worked hard to cope with her needs, but the results were not generally successful and the costs, both financially and emotionally, seemed exorbitant.

In presenting this story we have three separate but overlapping audiences in mind. Our primary audience is family members who will or who have already had to deal with all the angst and stress of being a caregiver. We offer lessons that we hope will help them. Another audience is those who oversee and work in the organizations and institutions that serve all these frail older persons. Some messages offer sympathy for their plight as they strive to do their best within all the perceived and real constraints they face; other messages are meant to push them to rethink their positions and their actions. Many underlying assumptions about what is feasible need to be reconsidered. Everyone acknowledges the general dissatisfaction with long-term care, but no one seems inclined to do something about it. This inertia is unacceptable. The final audience is the policy makers, those who pass legislation and develop rules. It is time to rethink the goals of long-term care and the system that has evolved to meet the needs of a growing segment of our population.

This tale should be a call to action for our nation. We operate a long-term care system that is a national disgrace. Every day thousands of people face situations similar to ours. Some are starting and others ending, but none has a happy story. The newcomers read how-to books in the hope that they can cram for a life crisis, but the problem lies not so much in their not knowing what to do (surely a geriatrician who does research on long-term care knows what to do) but in their being unable to get the care that is needed. The message is simple. The demands seem reasonable. The long-term care system should not be so hard to traverse. It should be more humane and more competent. One should not have to choose between quality of care and quality of life. One should be able to trust institutions to give the care they promise. The necessary personal care and the medical care should be coordinated.

Family members can and should do some things to protect their loved ones who are served by this imperfect system. But individual battles are David and Goliath matchups without the necessary divine intercession. A larger revolution is needed, one that can be supported by all our audiences. Few are happy with what today's long-term care system has become. Many of those most enmeshed in it, however, fear change because it may bring even worse conditions. We need to take a giant step back and recall what we are trying to accomplish. It will not come about through small adjustments. Big changes are needed.

The needed changes will not come easily. Our society has shown no interest in making anywhere near the investment in long-term care that we have made in acute care. We provide neither the technical competence nor the economic support that we offer in other areas. Part of the problem may be a basic sense of the futility of such care. What difference can good long-term care make? Although they are too often written off, good care can make all the difference in the lives of frail older people and their families.

We offer this story as both an inspiration and a challenge to all who will someday be looking for compassionate and effective long-term care for their parents or other elderly family members or for themselves. We offer some practical suggestions as well as some over-all recommendations about how to make the system work better. The frailty that comes with growing old can be traumatic enough without the care system's making it worse. Even with the best of care, growing old and frail can be heartbreaking. And so we hope this book will also assure you that you are not alone in your struggles.

We present our story first in chronological order. Then we go back to revisit certain aspects of care to comment on them in more depth from the perspective of the full experience. We realize that this organization may present some redundancy but we want to make sure that important points are clear. We conclude with a broad look at the long-term care system and the steps that individuals can take on their own and collectively to improve long-term care.

Background

To understand this story, you have to know a little about our mother. Ruth was an extremely attractive, intelligent woman with a certain elegance and panache about her. She had been married to a man who had achieved modest success as an executive in various men's retail clothing firms. He very much looked the part. Perhaps because clothing was our father's occupation and because our mother herself had been a showroom model, both of our parents had strong investments in their appearances. They made an elegant couple, always well dressed. They spent a great deal of time and money on their wardrobes. In 1959, however, our father lost his job and went into a series of downward spirals. During this period, Ruth, who had always been financially insecure and concerned about saving, became obsessed with the need to have a financial nest egg. Our father finally got back on his feet in 1965, when he and a partner opened a retail men's wear store in Manhattan. For the first time he was his own boss.

For the last five years of his life our parents were a happy couple. The years of financial insecurity gave way to a period of happy experiences: glamorous vacations and visits to grandchildren.

Our father died of a heart attack in September 1971 when he was fifty-nine years old. He had had a previous episode but seemed to have recovered. Ruth was left a widow at age fifty-six. She had not worked outside the home since their marriage in 1935. She was a high school graduate who had worked as a salesperson and model in a millinery wholesaler store until she married. Having essentially invested in our father's career for her married life, she decided, after an absence of thirty-six years, to try her hand in the labor market.

Her son-in-law helped her find a job using one her best skills: talking on the telephone. She became a supervisor for a national telephone-marketing firm. Unfortunately, her career as a working woman was brief; that job lasted only a few weeks. Her employers discovered she used the 800 line to call her family and friends all over the country rather than attending to business. (She liked to attribute her brief tenure to boredom, claiming she had quit the job. She never told us the true reason the job ended.) She did get a kick out of drawing unemployment insurance for a while, but that was her last foray into the business world.

Fortunately, Ruth had made some prudent investments and could live modestly off the income. She had few women friends and did not seek out the company of other women. After several months she began to go out on dates, much to the relief of Joan, who worried about her being alone and lonely. Men had always been attracted to Ruth and she certainly had not lost her charm or her appeal. Within a year after her husband's death she had two serious suitors.

Robert recalls:

I vividly remember coming back to New York with my wife for my father's one-year memorial service. It was a turning point in my relationship with my mother. She had arranged for us to meet (i.e., interview) her two suitors on consecutive nights. On the first evening, while she and my wife were getting ready I answered the doorbell. A rather elderly gentleman decked out in white trousers and a blue blazer was standing there with a bottle of scotch under his arm. He was my mother's date. I ushered him in and offered him a seat on the couch across from me to wait for the women. He sat with his hands in his lap. I had the image of a Norman Rockwell painting of the young boy coming to pick up his first date for the prom. I had to resist the temptation to ask him how school was. The tables had obviously turned. I was now the parental figure passing judgment on my mother's beaus. He finally said to me, "I want to assure you that I will take very good care of your mother." We went out to dinner and he and my mother danced while my wife and I sat as chaperones.

Ruth chose the other man, a retired pharmacist, whom we liked better too. They decided to move to Florida. They lived together for five years but never married. Obsessed with financial security, Ruth was careful to purchase the condominium in her name but let him share the monthly payments. Likewise she furnished it with a lot of things she brought from New York, but they shared the cost of any new furniture and the decoration of the apartment. This period was a high point in her life. They were an active couple. He pursued hobbies. She played bridge and golf and actually began attending adult education classes at a nearby university. But after a while she grew tired of him. Eventually she threw him out.

Ruth was one of two daughters. She maintained an intense rivalry with her sister, who was better off financially. Ruth felt that she had been poorly used by her sister, who failed to help her when Ruth was financially strapped. In the later years of their lives they rarely spoke, even though they both lived in the same town in Florida. Some years before Ruth became ill, her sister had a severe stroke, which left her very dependent. Ruth did not visit her on her own, partly because of the long-standing animosity, partly because of her aversion to disability. When Robert visited his mother, he would occasionally also see his aunt, even though it seemed like a breach of loyalty. On one occasion, he was able to persuade Ruth to go with him. She came away in tears. She was shocked by her sister's appearance. Even though her sister had round-the-clock help that allowed her to live in a luxurious condominium, it was obvious that she derived little pleasure from her daily existence. This experience left Ruth even more convinced that she never wanted to be disabled.

Over the next decade she had several romantic involvements, including one with a much younger man, a lawyer who had come to visit his mother in the same condominium complex. Ruth loved the image of herself as a swinger. Indeed, one night she called Robert and after a general conversation quietly asked him about the symptoms of venereal disease. Although she was a little embarrassed, she was also obviously a little pleased about how this question would add to her image. She did turn out to have a mild case of a sexually transmitted parasite.

Later she had a tempestuous affair with a man about ten years older than she. He had sophisticated tastes and introduced her to a world of culture and unworried wealth. She was devoted to him for several years and even nursed him through his dependency resulting from hip surgery, but she eventually left him after she discovered he was seeing another woman. That was probably the last great love of her life. Afterward, she seemed to lose interest in dating. Sadly, she also stopped attending classes and playing duplicate bridge because her former lover still attended the bridge club. The only activity she kept up was her walk in her condo swimming pool. She would go late in the afternoon almost every day. Even then she managed to make herself the center of attention. She generated a major dispute because she tended to do her pool walking topless. One of the neighbors complained, and she reveled in her negotiations with the condo board over the incident.

Overall, Ruth had managed to create an independent life for herself. Before the swimming pool controversy she served as the president of her condominium and was a force to be reckoned with. She alienated many people with her direct style and had few close friends, always preferring the company of men. She worked so hard at the job that she effectively made the manger's position unnecessary. However, she was also very domineering and suffered others' opinions poorly. She made decisions about the building unilaterally and acted without consultation. Ultimately she antagonized many of the other residents and they voted her out. She saw Joan and her children very frequently. Robert was living in California and later in Minnesota during those years and her visits to him were infrequent, typically around special occasions. More often people came to her. She liked to be on her own turf. She could tolerate sharing her space only on a limited basis and was very much a creature of her own routines.

When she did visit family, she always arrived with a magnificent wardrobe. When children and grandchildren visited her, she made gifts to them of the clothing she had tired of, and it seemed to give her genuine pleasure to share the items, as well as to clear the way for more. She continued to have a high interest in fashion, maintaining and storing her clothing, shoes, and accessories with exquisite care.

She also had a strong desire for privacy. She hated sharing a bathroom when she traveled, in part because she had full dentures and never wanted anyone to see her without them in place.

Ruth's preference for the company of men extended even to her children. She loved to go out to eat when Robert visited but was reluctant to go out to nice restaurants with Joan, for fear of their looking like two women without escorts. She preferred to shop, go the beach, and go to movies when Joan came.

She had a few close friends but strove never to be beholden to anyone. Ruth had one very close friend and neighbor in the condo, whose untimely death was a huge blow to her. Apparently, the two women had made a pact to assist each other to die if and when either one became incapacitated. This woman was one of the only friends we never heard our mother criticize.

Ruth was much happier giving aid or doing favors than accepting them. She befriended strangers in need of help and even established what passed for close friendships with people who worked in service occupations, such as dry cleaners and hair stylists. She spent the later years of her life in a fairly solitary mode. She would speak to neighbors freely but rarely sought the company of others, save her family.

Joan repeatedly broached the subject of Ruth's moving from Florida to New York to be near her, but each time the response was adamantly negative. Ruth valued her autonomy very highly. She made it very clear that she did not want to live in the north unless she became ill or disabled. Even under those conditions, she would want to be near Joan but not "on top of her."

Gradually, Ruth began showing signs of aging. To relieve long-standing problems with cataracts she had a lens implant but never recovered her vision in one eye, despite a subsequent corneal transplant. Nonetheless, she continued to drive and retain her independence.

We noticed some signs of memory failure, but it was not clear just how serious the lapses were. Ruth certainly enjoyed having the same conversations over and over, most of which were reminiscences of various times in her life. She talked a great deal about our father and about her own father. She seemed to be trying to retell her life story to give it more meaning and improve her role. Although she had had bitter fights with our father and had been frustrated with his inability to push himself forward aggressively, he now emerged as a shining hero. She talked a lot about her youth and her relations with her own father, whom she adored. She maintained her running feud with her sister, fueled by recollections of their youth and the years when our father was unemployed and exacerbated by the events surrounding the decision to put her father in a nursing home. This memory was particularly painful to her. She tried hard to place much of the onus on her sister but clearly felt guilty for ever allowing the decision to be made.

Eventually, especially once her last romance ended, she seemed to adopt the life-style of a person with no social life. She stayed up late at night and slept very late in the mornings. This pattern of late rising was not new. When we were growing up we never saw our mother before noon. The near absence of a social life did not mean Ruth had lost interest in life. She read *Vanity Fair* regularly and gossiped with her granddaughter about the articles. She avidly watched television news panel and interview shows, especially Charlie Rose. She identified closely with glamorous women like Jacqueline Kennedy and Lauren

Bacall. But her world was contracting. She entertained less. She had fewer occasions to wear her clothes and hence less reason to shop for them. Driving became more difficult.

Gradually a series of chronic diseases began to take their toll. One rare routine physical exam revealed a breast mass. Ruth was adamant that she would not have surgery. Even the entreaties of her physician son had no effect. She would rather be dead than disfigured. About six months later she was found to have an abnormal pap smear. We finally talked her into having a simple biopsy, which showed a carcinoma in situ, a very treatable level of cervical cancer. But once again she refused any surgery. She argued that she would outlive both cancers, a prophecy that proved true.

Ruth had never tolerated pain well. On the several occasions she had chest or stomach pains her first reaction was to call 911. Over the course of six months, she called 911 at least six times and wound up in an emergency room each time. As a result, this woman who all her life had avoided doctors became a frequent visitor to the emergency room. Each encounter generated a great deal of expense and anxiety. Most of them proved to be false alarms. But on one occasion she was found to have suffered a mild heart attack. The cardiologist insisted on a cardiac catheterization procedure to view the status of her coronary arteries. When Robert responded that this procedure was warranted only as a prelude to coronary artery surgery, which she had already refused, the cardiologist replied that he still could not care for her without knowing the status of her coronary arteries. In the end Ruth's attachment to the cardiologist triumphed. Rather than lose a doctor she liked, she agreed to the procedure, despite her fears about it. As it turned out, her arteries were fine.

The signs of memory loss became more and more evident. Ruth would get lost driving in familiar places. Once, for example, when

Joan was with her she could not find the storefront of the dry cleaner she frequented. As it turned out, they had been within yards, but the entrance was recessed slightly from the main road. Periodically she would call Joan and complain that her mind was not right, that she could tell that she was "losing it."

For a while we thought that these lapses in memory might be related to her increased drinking. Although Ruth had never been a heavy drinker, she had begun consuming substantial quantities of wine and later of vodka. When Robert realized what was happening, he spoke to her about the problem and she actually gave up drinking almost entirely. But the memory problems did not improve.

Although we questioned whether she should be driving and she had considered selling her car, she continued to drive up to the day before she had the stroke. She wanted to live on her own and seemed to be able to manage fairly well.

Because Ruth was calling 911 so often and showing signs of cognitive impairment, however, we decided to hire a local case manager. Although one of us visited her at least every other month, and Joan spoke with her once a day or more, we thought it important that Ruth form a relationship with someone close by who could become a point of first contact in an emergency and help manage her life and address her anxiety. A case manager could also look in on her to make sure she was getting along all right.

The practice of hiring case managers as local, surrogate family members has been growing in this country for at least a decade. Families living many miles away from older parents who have retired to the Sunbelt become anxious about their parents' well-being. Under long-distance case management, the case managers can help relieve that anxiety by overseeing and assisting as needed and communicating the situation back to the families. We began our search by calling a woman who has made a national reputation as one of the founders of this movement to explain our situation and see what she could offer. She agreed to put one of her staff on the case. We quickly discovered that surrogate care management is indeed a business and it is not cheap. Not only was the hourly rate high (about one hundred dollars even after our "professional discount") but the organization required a deposit of several hundred dollars.

The case management agency director wisely chose a male social worker as the case manager and, after we introduced the idea, Ruth agreed to see him. Our goal was to have the case manager establish a relationship such that he would be Ruth's first point of contact. We expected him to do an assessment, establish a relationship through periodic contact, and then be available whenever help was needed.

The first report from the case manager (accompanied by a bill) indicated that he was getting to know our mother and she was telling him the stories of her life. As we talked with Ruth it became clear that she saw him as a friendly visitor but never as someone to help her. He made several more visits and learned even more about her, but she kept calling 911 or one of us when she had a problem. It quickly became clear that Ruth would not be managed by a case manager. She wanted the real thing. She wanted attention from her family.

The case manager, we learned, never did develop an effective rapport that would have made him a natural point of contact. He did not really try to form a therapeutic alliance with Ruth. He never went with her to a doctor or rehearsed what to do in an emergency. Since we were paying the bills, the company considered us the client and the case manager seemed more concerned about sending us reports after each visit than with developing a trusting relationship with Ruth. Indeed, he was somewhat patronizing about her as a decision maker.

It proved hard to explain to the company that we were not looking for a James Bond to spy on our mother and tell us what we already knew. We were looking for someone to bond with her. Perhaps because the case management agency knew Robert by reputation and knew his wife quite well, they focused their efforts on us out of a desire to impress; unfortunately they did it the wrong way.

Ruth's dread of becoming disabled was likely influenced in large measure by a the devastating experience she had had with nursing-home care when she participated in admitting her father to what was meant to be a short stay in a nursing home prior to Joan's wedding. He became so despondent there that he tried to kill himself and died soon after of complications of his illness. The scar of that experience never left her. The last thing she wanted was to become a nursing-home resident. And it was the last thing her children wanted for her as well.

LESSONS

1   An intense desire to maintain independence is common among older persons, who fear becoming a burden on their children. For many, too, the opportunity to leave a financial legacy makes them loath to spend money on themselves, even for supportive care.

2   One of the greatest challenges in working with older people, especially family members, is handling the moment when they can no longer drive safely because of poor eyesight or memory. Taking away a person's car is traumatizing because it renders the person dependent on others. The financial advantage of taking taxis rather than maintaining a car cannot offset the change in status and life-style that giving up one's car represents.

3   Older people often have a strong sense of what is important in their health care, and few people have difficulty recognizing an older person's preferences. Problems often arise, however, in finding ways to honor those preferences.

4   Making realistic advance plans for long-term care is difficult. While one can identify general approaches to take, the confrontation with reality may be quite different from the ideas raised in theory.

5   Long-distance case management may be an answer for some people, but not all. Before hiring a case manager, however, it is important to consider the goals and the costs and to remember that because the children generally pay for the service, they become the de facto client rather than the older person. The task should be to provide support to the frail older person, especially in negotiating the complex health system, not to provide information for their children. Ideally case managers could assist older people to negotiate the complex health care system more efficiently and to achieve the ends the older persons wanted to achieve.

6   Older people probably think a lot about their parents and siblings as they contemplate their own old age.

7   The onset of health problems is insidious. It is even harder to detect change when you are not there to observe it yourself. Long-distance family members—even those with the sophistication of a geriatrician—have great difficulty detecting change, especially when they must rely on reports from the person affected. And those living near or with an older person may be less sensitive to change that is gradual than are those who visit intermittently and get periodic snapshots.

The Stroke

On May 17, 1999, our eighty-five-year-old mother woke up confused and with a headache. Her right side was weak. This time she did not call 911. Instead, for reasons we will never understand, and with abilities we will never know how she summoned, she dragged herself out of her condominium apartment, into the elevator, and out onto the floor of the building's lobby. She was able to raise her arm and signal the condo handyman, who was on his "rounds." He had a relative who had suffered a stroke and immediately deduced what had happened and called an ambulance. Meanwhile a neighbor called Joan, who then called Robert.

We both got on planes and headed to Boca Raton. The person we found in the intensive care unit (ICU) looked like a little old lady. Her dentures had been removed. The right side of her body was paralyzed. Her speech was slurred and almost incomprehensible.

Ruth was admitted to intensive care because her physicians wanted to monitor her closely. This hospital did not have a dedicated stroke unit. Intensive care means just that. The ratio of nursing staff is higher than on a regular hospital unit. Because patients who are kept there need close attention, it is a busy place, in motion twenty-four hours a day. Such a busy place can be very disturbing for someone who is already confused by both a catastrophic disease and the sudden change in venue. In some forms of torture, prisoners are put in brightly lit, noisy rooms and forced to stay awake. The ICU was like this. The lights never went off. The undertone of activity-associated noise was constant. Thus, the price for active attention is continuous overstimulation and confusion.

As a result of the stroke, Ruth was aphasic, that is, she could not speak effectively, and our efforts to communicate with her in writing proved futile. She was extremely irritable and agitated. It seemed impossible for her to get comfortable. Despite her aphasia she was able to indicate over and again that she wanted her sheets smoothed. We could never get them right. No matter how many hours we stayed near her, the moment we left, she would scream for us and express her concerns that we were abandoning her. This fear of being left in the strange setting was a theme that would reoccur with many of her subsequent hospitalizations.

Ruth reacted very badly to her new condition. It is hard to say how much was the direct effect of the stroke and how much was influenced by the environment. For whatever reason, she became very agitated and restless. Despite not being able to articulate, however, she had no problem conveying her intentions. Without being able to raise her voice, she yelled at everyone, especially us. She constantly complained (largely by gesture) that her bedclothes needed to be straightened (and once they were straightened she would proceed immediately to toss around and mess them up and complain all over again). She was irritable and aggressive with the staff and with us.

Undoubtedly she was frightened. She did not know exactly what had happened, though she could relate (in her unclear speech) the story of what she had done to get to the apartment lobby. She now found herself in exactly the predicament she most feared. She was severely disabled and absolutely dependent. Her response was aggression.

The neurologist looking after her wanted to keep her in the ICU because of the need to monitor her blood pressure, which was now high for the first time in her life, probably as a result of the stroke. The first day or so was spent stabilizing her medical condition. The CAT scan showed a clear area of hemorrhage, which mapped well against her neurological loss. The stroke was not totally unexpected, given her medical condition. She had a history of periodic episodes of atrial fibrillation, a form of rapid heart beat. These episodes usually converted to a normal rhythm spontaneously. This condition is associated with a danger of small blood clots breaking off from the heart and going to the brain, and the usual treatment is anticoagulation. Indeed, Ruth had been anticoagulated at various periods over the past several years, but it was difficult for her to be maintained at the right level. She bruised herself badly several times and eventually the anticoagulation was discontinued. Likely during such an episode of fibrillation she had launched a blood clot to her brain, which created a blockage in the blood vessels in her brain and bleeding at the same time.

Despite the need to stabilize and monitor her, keeping her in the ICU proved to be a high price to pay for the modest nursing attention she received. The environment was too active and the last thing Ruth needed in her confused condition was more stimulation. Although there were many nurses, their priorities lay with patients whose conditions were less stable.

The doctors were attentive, but their attention spans were short. Once Ruth's condition stabilized she was no longer an interesting case. Her persistent agitation caused some concern. The doctors were not sure whether it represented an expansion of her stroke or some other reaction to the situation. Her having a son who was a physician, especially a geriatrician, was a mixed blessing. Robert was strongly tempted to make suggestions but felt the need to be diplomatic. Ruth had two doctors: a cardiologist and a neurologist, but these two doctors never met; they communicated through the chart. As a result, in effect, one hand never knew just what the other was doing. Robert tried not to be directive or to point out inconsistencies in care that were not life threatening. (Nothing of that magnitude occurred.) Despite some anxieties about the care that was being provided, Robert never intervened actively. He did not press to transfer Ruth to a less frenetic ward because he too believed she needed the attention she was getting and the ability for the staff to act quickly in case of an emergency.

One example of the lack of direct communication between the doctors is the duplication of tests to re-evaluate Ruth's stroke status. Because she was not recovering as well as we had hoped, the neurologist decided to order another CAT scan. Somehow, on the same day she received that second CAT scan, she also received an MRI (magnetic resonance imaging), a test that offered little new information over and above the CAT scan. Both tests are very expensive. Doing both was wasteful.

We never found out why she was given both tests. Perhaps the neurologist ordered one and the cardiologist the other. Our previous experiences with the health care system in Florida left us with the impression that Florida doctors like to give tests, even when the ostensible reason for giving them is unclear. This fondness does not seem to be driven by greed. The doctors who ordered the tests did not perform them and did not derive any revenue from them. Nor did the hospital benefit. Under Medicare the hospital was paid a fixed amount for our mother's stay regardless of how many tests were performed. Thus, this practice cost the hospital money, especially when redundant tests were ordered that would not affect the care. We had the sense that such tests seemed to offer some misplaced appearance of protection against lawsuits brought in response to oversights.

Every new crisis reinforced our observation that doctors really speak in meaningful ways only to other doctors. Thus, from the first moment Joan arrived at the hospital, she was grateful that Robert was there to talk with the doctors. He was better able than she to understand what the doctors were saying and to make informed decisions. This is not to say that we did not encounter some very thoughtful, well-intentioned doctors along the journey, but our experience made it clear that doctors prefer to deal directly with other members of their profession.

Medicine is at best a matter of guesswork and those patients who do not follow the "normal" progression or pattern of their illnesses are both an annoyance and a puzzlement. Medicine is frequently called an art or a "practice," but it is not a perfected art. The meaning of that phrase became more and more apparent with our mother's case. As the week in ICU progressed, we felt that many of the care decisions that were made were based on judgments and not certainty. Some of them were wrong. Also in those first days we began a long and wrenching effort, which is dealt with in later chapters, to separate our mother's behavior from the person we used to know, love, and trust.

In addition to the comfort of having Robert there to speak with and understand the doctors, Joan felt lucky to have his support. Looking back, she realized she was in shock for the entire first week after the stroke. Knowing her brother was there enabled her to shut down in some ways and let him be "in charge" and on top of things that first week She did not begin to fully process everything until he left to return home and she was the one in charge of overseeing Ruth's recovery. At that point, as is human nature, Joan was able because of necessity to rise to the occasion.

Soon after Robert left, the doctors found themselves in a dilemma. Ruth's agitation was making it hard to manage her. She was constantly pulling out her intravenous (IV) lines and pulling off her monitoring wires. They restrained her by literally tying her up, a practice that is generally considered unacceptable . They wanted to sedate her but feared doing so because her level of consciousness was an important indication of the condition of her stroke. A few days after her stoke, when the doctors did try to sedate her they discovered that the sedatives had a paradoxical effect. After initially calming her, the sedatives then made her more excitable.

Although more nurses were on duty in the ICU than on a regular ward, they were usually harried and few had the time (or the inclination) to simply sit with Ruth and try to reassure her. That was our job. It was a tough job. It was boring and also painful. Not only did we have to constantly observe our mother reduced to this pitiful state, but she would lash out at us as if to blame us for getting her into it. After a couple of days Ruth's condition seemed to stabilize, though her agitated behavior did not improve. Nonetheless, the hospital began to press for a discharge plan, and a discharge planner came to see us to discuss post-hospital care. Hospitals try to keep stays as short as possible because, under Medicare rules, they are paid a set amount for care regardless of how long the patient actually stays. (If a patient requires an inordinately long stay, the hospital does receive an additional payment, but these cases are rare.) Also, the discharge planner is a hospital employee, usually a nurse or a social worker, whose job is to help the patient and her family arrange for care after she leaves the hospital. But because of the Medicare system of paying hospitals a fixed amount of money for each hospital stay, the discharge planner is under great pressure to identify plans that can be implemented immediately.

The hospital's interests may thus run counter to the patient's and the family's. Moreover, making good decisions in these circumstances can be quite time consuming and complex. Before a plan can be made there must be some level of consensus about what outcomes the post-hospital care should be attempting to achieve. For example, is the first concern safety or the patient's ability to live independently? How much medical and functional recovery can be realistically expected? What modes of care are most likely to produce the desired outcomes? Once a general approach to care is chosen, the next step is to choose the provider of that care. In our case, that step was complex. We first had to decide whether to look for a facility in Florida or in Long Island near Joan or in Minneapolis near Robert.

These decisions may take some time to make. In many cases family must first be assembled. Once together, rarely does everyone agree about the goals of care or the best location to provide it. Most older patients want to go home, even when data suggest that they will fare better medically in more supervised surroundings. The sense of urgency imposed by the hospital rarely allows adequate time to resolve all the conflicts. Furthermore, the discharge planner, who is actually the hospital's advocate, is likely to propose the most expeditious solution. This person, who should be facilitating the discussion, may be more anxious to conclude it.

We were fortunate, going into the meeting with the discharge planner, that we had already accomplished several of the essential elements in decision making. As Ruth's only immediate family, we were together and in agreement about our goals. Our emphasis was on maximizing Ruth's functional recovery. Given her condition, Ruth was not an active part of the decision process. We were also fortunate to have our own expertise. Ironically, Robert's research included work in discharge planning and post-hospital care, especially for conditions like stroke. That work had shown that the discharge plans under study were usually badly made. Insufficient time had been allowed for considering the options and just what form of care was likely to achieve the best results. Little time had been allowed for families to gather and resolve their different feelings about placement. Different viewpoints, including different agendas for the patient and her family, were often left unreconciled. In the case of stroke, the nature of post-hospital care made a big difference in patients' functional recovery. Patients discharged to so-called skilled nursing facilities (nursing homes) did not do as well those sent to rehabilitation units or even those sent home with home health care.

We were left to consider what was the next best step. The basic options were a formal rehabilitation program, rehabilitation in a skilled nursing facility, going home with home care, or just going home with no formal care. We determined that Ruth needed an active course of rehabilitation. The big question was where. Robert's knowledge of the field made us reluctant to consider a skilled nursing facility.

The idea that Ruth could enter an inpatient rehabilitation program in Florida on her own seemed untenable. Even if she could and the rehabilitation went well, we recognized that we would still be faced with the question of what would happen when she was ready for discharge. Furthermore, it seemed unlikely that she would emerge from rehabilitation without substantial residual dependency. Her poor social support system made it especially unlikely that she could manage well on her own. We could hire someone to look after her, but we would then be totally dependent on a stranger supervised from afar. The more we thought about the situation, the clearer it became that this was the time to think about making a permanent geographical move. She would go either to Long Island to be near Joan or to Minneapolis to be near Robert.

For a lot of reasons we decided on Long Island. Even though Robert most likely could arrange and monitor rehabilitation better because of his expertise and his place in the medical community, Joan could not accept the idea that her mother would be in Minnesota and she would be in New York, and Robert knew Joan would be solicitous and very much present. He also recognized that he would not be able to sustain the same attention temperamentally or logistically, especially given the busy travel schedule he and his wife maintained. Moreover, Ruth had made it abundantly clear that if she were ever incapacitated to the point where she could not stay in Florida, she wanted to be in New York.

Making decisions in these moments of crisis set in play a series of events that would have major repercussions. We knew that the pressure of time and the emotional turmoil that accompany serious illness make rational decision-making difficult and frankly unusual but that given the enormity of the implications these decisions should be made carefully. We therefore tried hard to think through the long-term implications of the possible alternatives. Once we had decided that our mother would not likely be able to function on her own, we had crossed a Rubicon. If she were no longer able to remain in Florida on her own, even with personal assistance, we knew she had to be transported to live near one of us. Knowledge of our dispositions and our mother's predilections made the final choice about which of us she would live near relatively easy.

We could have postponed this final decision if we had decided on rehabilitative care in Florida, but such care would have required oversight by one of us. It would have meant that at least one of us would have had to take even more time away from a demanding job. Moreover, there was no reason to believe that we would be in any more certain position after rehabilitation. True, we would have a better sense of how much function Ruth had regained, but neither believed that she would ever again be able to live on her own.

At the same time, the decision to move Ruth out of Florida meant that she no longer had a household. Any future decisions that involved her living in the community would involve building a household from scratch. Even the cost of moving her furniture would likely be prohibitive.

Although we had decided to move Ruth to New York rather than to Minnesota for rehabilitation, we had not yet made any clear plans about what would happen after she left rehabilitation. Moving her to Joan's house even to recuperate and buy some time was not an option. The house was too small to accommodate Ruth, and it had many stairs and only one full bathroom. Moreover, the idea of the two of them living under the same roof did not sit well with any of us as a permanent plan.

Our decision-making had the advantage that one of us was professionally involved in studying just this process, even though he was emotionally entangled in the present case. Most people facing this dilemma have no such resource. In theory, the persons best positioned to help with these decisions are the hospital discharge planners; but they are under great pressure to move patients out quickly. Given that motivation, discharge planners tend to view the first train leaving the station as the best one regardless of its destination.

Making these decisions is complex and should be separated into two distinct steps. The first step is to decide what kind of care is likely to bring about the best outcome. In our mother's case this question seemed simple. The major goal was as much functional improvement as possible. Research data suggests that persons sent to organized rehabilitation units do better than those who go to nursing homes.

The second step is to decide which facility of the general type selected—in our case, a rehabilitation center—can provide the best care under the circumstances. At this stage location becomes a major issue, and once we had decided that Ruth should go to Long Island to be near Joan, we set about finding out which facilities had the best reputation for effective rehabilitation. At this stage, because rehabilitation facilities are more like hospitals and are not intended for long-stay residence, we were less concerned about ambiance and amenities than effectiveness in improving functioning.

Once the location decision was made, we had to make a series of complex arrangements. We needed to find a rehabilitation unit that would accept Ruth and we needed to organize transportation. Again Robert's institutional connections made our process easier; he called his geriatric colleagues in New York to inquire about good units. They recommended one near Joan on Long Island. He called the medical director and explained the medical situation. They had no openings but expected a discharge in a few days that would create a slot.

Most people facing this dilemma will not have professional contacts. They will have to rely on the discharge planners. These hospital resources can provide lists of places but they may vary widely in the extent of their actual knowledge about the potential locations. There is no systematic guide to rehabilitation units. (The homepage of the Centers for Medicare and Medicaid Services provides some information about nursing homes; see Appendix 2.)

The next big question was how to get Ruth from Boca Raton, Florida, to Glen Cove, Long Island. The answer was an air ambulance. The hospital discharge planner was already distressed because our complicated arrangements threatened to lengthen Ruth's hospital stay. She gave us a list of air ambulance companies but declined to play an active role in either recommending one or helping make the arrangements. We got on the phone.

It turned out that air ambulance service is a competitive business. It is probably also quite lucrative because the prices were steep (over nine thousand dollars) and not covered by Medicare. But there was considerable variation in those prices. We identified one that seemed to be in the lower range (but by no means inexpensive) and received some reassurance from the discharge planner that the company we chose had been reliable in the past. Like all charters, the company strives to avoid down time or empty plane time. They sought to schedule our trip so it would fit into their already scheduled trips. We had to balance our timing needs with theirs. Availability thus became an important consideration in our selection of a company.

The requirements were extensive. In addition to the two-person crew, an EMT (emergency medical technician) was needed to oversee Ruth's care during the trip. The company warned us that the plane was barely big enough to hold Ruth on a stretcher along with this crew, but we insisted on accompanying her. We needed conventional ambulances at both ends: one to take her from the Florida hospital to the airfield and another to take her from the Long Island airfield to the rehabilitation hospital. Fortunately, the air ambulance company arranged for the other ambulances. We were now into a juggling act.

We booked a tentative time for the air ambulance, assuming a bed would open at the rehabilitation hospital. When we called back to the rehabilitation hospital they said they would have a bed available on Friday afternoon, but we had to arrive before three o'clock because the rehabilitation hospital would have much less staff on the upcoming weekend and would not accept new admissions then.

We confirmed with the air ambulance company and explained the time constraint. They said they would pick up our mother at 8:00 A.M. sharp. She needed to be ready with all her information and release forms. We contacted the discharge planner, who agreed to get the information ready and organize the discharge. Ruth's neurologist agreed to the discharge plan. Everything seemed to be in order.

On Thursday night the neurologist signed the discharge orders. We got the discharging physician to prepare a discharge summary that we could take with us because we knew the transfer of information between a hospital and the next point along the line was usually poor. We spoke with the night nurses at the Florida hospital to ask especially that they not sedate Ruth even if she was agitated because she responded poorly to the medication. They promised to try to communicate that information to the day shift. We left the hospital at around 11:00 P.M. to pack for the trip to New York, thinking everything was finally under control. Little did we know.

When we arrived at the hospital at seven o'clock on Friday morning we found Ruth fast asleep. She did not seem ready for discharge. The nurse cheerfully explained that Ruth had become very agitated during the night and especially since she was going to have a long plane ride, they had given her an injection of Ativan (a sedative) to calm her. This was the very action we had worked so hard to avoid, because Ruth had already shown a strong negative reaction to such medications.

The ambulance crew showed up right on time but they explained that they could take only one passenger in the ambulance besides the patient. The other one would have to follow in a cab. Joan went with Ruth and Robert took the cab. The ambulance crew gave him the name of the private airfield where the air ambulance was parked. Unfortunately, it turned out to be the wrong field. After Robert arrived and dismissed the cab, he discovered that the air ambulance was actually at the other end of town at another private field. Because it was so critical that we arrive within the window the receiving hospital had dictated, this became a crisis. One of the mechanics finally agreed to drive Robert to the other field. We got on board and settled in.

Joan had felt especially unglued as the ambulance took off, fearing that Robert would not make it to the airport in time to fly with them to New York. When she got to the airstrip, she pressed the pilot to wait for Robert, which fortunately he did. Joan felt overwhelmed by the task of moving our mother all that way. She placed heavy reliance on Robert, expecting that he would know what to do. In truth, no one anticipated just how tumultuous that flight would be. We came to view it as a metaphor for the entire disruption we were about to impose on our mother's life.

On the plane, as Ruth began to wake up she became very agitated. Confused and disoriented, she flailed about wildly, pulling at her IVs and moaning. All efforts to reassure her were of no avail. She could not understand where she was and indeed the tiny space was like nothing she had seen before. The Ativan only made things worse. There we were, twenty thousand feet in the air in a small jet plane with a seemingly crazy woman thrashing about on a narrow stretcher in a very confined space, pulling at her IVs and raving. We all took turns trying to calm her: Robert, Joan, and the EMT. No one was very effective. Finally the EMT insisted on giving her more sedative. She fell asleep.

The sadness and irony of this situation did not elude us. Our mother, who had worried her whole life about money and was so averse to any extravagance but who so appreciated luxury and status, could not even enjoy her only ride on a private Lear jet.

Another ambulance and Joan's husband met the plane. Robert rode with the ambulance and the others rode on ahead to the hospital. Our heavily sedated mother whom we delivered to the rehabilitation doctor was, for all intents and purposes, comatose. The physiatrist (rehabilitation doctor) looked at Robert as if he were not the son and a fellow physician but a used-car salesman who had just sold him a lemon. This was certainly not the patient he had agreed to accept over the telephone.

To be covered by Medicare, a patient in a rehabilitation hospital must demonstrate the potential for improvement as a result of reha-bilitation and be able to physically endure at least three hours a day of active rehabilitative therapy (i.e., physical therapy, occupational therapy, or speech therapy). At that point, our mother did not seem like a very strong candidate. Fortunately, no one has ever defined just what a day means. In many rehabilitation units, it refers only to week-days. The down time meant that Ruth would have a chance to recover over the weekend.

Looking back on this episode and all the things that went wrong, we are amazed that we pulled it off. We could not have done what we did, however, if we had not taken over all the decision making. Some might argue that the price was too high. Our mother was effectively reduced to an object about whom decisions were made. We could have taken more active steps to engage her in the decision process. We did not believe, however, given her physical and cognitive state, that her opinions were rational. We felt that she could not appreciate the circumstances and the consequences of alternative actions. Nonetheless, we decided that without even giving her the chance to try. It is unlikely that her subsequent confusion was a result of this one-sided process, but we will never know.

Even when Ruth did have occasional periods of lucidity during her hospital stay, it was not clear that she appreciated the limitations of her abilities and her prognosis. Like almost every other older patient, she expressed a strong desire to return home. And like most families of the afflicted, we viewed that preference as illogical. Once we decided that she needed to go to Long Island to be near Joan, however, she seemed to acquiesce.

Ruth did indeed have occasional periods of lucidity. At one point in the Florida hospital stay she recalled that several weeks earlier, before her stroke, she and Robert had gone shopping to purchase a new outfit for her to wear to his daughter's wedding, which was just a few weeks off. Ever the prudent shopper, she insisted that he take back the outfit for credit since she would not be able to attend the wedding.

Our taking over the decision making for Ruth effectively set the pattern for subsequent acts. We had crossed a silent threshold to where we were now the parental figures evaluating the situation and taking actions. We might make efforts to involve our mother in some decisions but this was no longer a democracy, nor was she a sovereign state.

The discharge process was distressing for all of us. The hospital staff did little to make it easier. Once we elected to move outside the regular process, which would have entailed making a transfer to a local rehabilitation center, the hospital's concern and the concern of all health personnel was directed largely at facilitating the move as quickly as possible.

LESSONS

1   Intensive Care Units are good for patients who need intensive care, but they may have serious drawbacks too. Although doctors are inclined to use ICUs because the patients get more attention, intensive care may not always be the best care for everyone. ICUs are especially poor places to treat confused older people, and data is emerging to suggest that they are associated with poorer results for stroke patients. Family members may find it difficult to oppose a doctor's decision to put an older patient in an ICU, but they need to be very observant about how such a setting might be making the situation worse and willing to raise such possibilities with the medical staff.

2   Hospitalizations are upsetting at the best of times; hospitals are dangerous places to treat confused older people. Families need to recognize that bad things can happen and be very vigilant.

3   Hospitals still use physical restraints, though nursing homes have largely stopped using them. Institutions dedicated to active treatment tend to be insensitive to the effects of restraints on the person receiving them.

4   Sedatives and other psychoactive medications (e.g., Haldol, Ativan) may have both more profound effects and more paradoxical effects (e.g., agitating them rather than quieting them) on older people.

5   Every institution has its own way of doing things. Few procedures are designed to make the patients' lives more comfortable. Hospital routines are designed for the convenience of the staff, not the patients and their families, and no amount of advocacy is likely to change that fact.

6   Do not trust the hospital to do the right things. Their interests may
       be different from yours. Even the doctors may not always have
       the patient's (or the family's) best interests at heart. They may be
       under various pressures to move patients out or just be in a hurry
       and want to do what is easiest. You need to be willing to take
       on authority figures, to question, and to report changes that seem
       important.

7   Do not assume that information will be effectively transferred
       from one shift to the next. You need to be proactive in pointing
       out changes in the patient's condition that shift workers may not
       see.

8   Being a pest, particularly a hypervigilant pest, will not endear
       you to the staff. You have to walk a fine line between being at-
       tentive and assertive and being so aggressive as to alienate the
       very people you depend on to provide help.

9   Older people are regularly left out of the decision-making pro-
       cess. The more urgent the issue, the less older people's prefer-
       ences are considered. Their preferences for going home, espe-
       cially, are discounted as unrealistic. Furthermore, the underlying
       principles, such as a desire for control or a reluctance to be a
       burden, may also be overlooked. Family members must struggle
       with their new role as surrogate decision makers while they try
       to act as advocates for their loved ones. If they do not press to
       involveolder patients in the decisions, it is unlikely they will be
       involved. Sometimes the pressure and complexities of the deci-
       sions seem just too great to go through the painful and often slow
       process of getting an older person to express an opinion. And
       then when the opinion expressed (usually to go home) does not
       seem realistic and is contrary to what the family thinks is best, it
       can raise feelings of guilt.

10   A hospital may say that its rush to discharge a patient is provoked
       by Medicare rules. That is only partially true. Medicare pays
       hospitals a fixed amount for every patient admitted (the amount
       varies with the diagnosis). Thus, hospitals make more money

on shorter admissions. But patients have rights and can appeal discharge decisions. Most families need an advocate to fight such a battle. The discharge planner is a hospital employee and therefore not a good advocate in such a situation. The best approach may be to hire a lawyer, preferably one with experience in these sorts of battles.

11   The discharge planner's job is to move patients out as quickly as possible. Your job is to make the best decision possible under the circumstances. Making good discharge plans is difficult and takes time. The first available discharge location may not be the best one. Therefore, when a hospital pushes for a discharge, you need to push back and exert your right to make an informed, deliberate decision.

12   Over and above the emotional stress, the feelings of fear, guilt, and anxiety, and the pressure to act quickly is the difficulty of obtaining adequate information about post-discharge options and their relative effectiveness. The first question to be addressed is, What kind of care will produce the best results? For example, is a formal rehabilitation hospital better than a nursing home or home health care? The next question is, Which specific place among those that offer the desired type of care can best fulfill the family's goals for the patient? That question raises a different set of issues, such as convenience, atmosphere, and technical competence.

13   The first available location may not be the best one. The discharge planner may be able to give you good information, but you need to question the basis for any suggestion and whether the planner has firsthand knowledge. Also, be aware that the discharge planner may try to pressure you into taking the easiest route, usually a nursing home.

14   How-to books and Web sites can help in the search for appropriate places for elderly post-discharge patients (see Appendixes 1 and 2). You also may want to consult an independent case manager to act as facilitator. Even though this step costs money,

it can have big pay-offs, financially and personally. Do not be afraid to ask for the time you need.

15   The immediate decisions made in the heat of the moment will shape all subsequent decisions. Despite the pressures to act quickly, try to think carefully and deliberately. Write down the options and the goals you are trying to maximize. Family members may not necessarily have the same goals, and some may be reluctant to express their feelings about ultimate goals. Nonetheless, families will never agree on a strategy if they do not agree on the goals.

Rehabilitation

The rehabilitation doctor was clearly distressed when he saw our mother, hardly looking like a patient ready for active rehabilitation, Nonetheless, he admitted her late on Friday afternoon.

Ordinarily a late Friday admission is wasteful because full rehabilitation cannot be mustered over the weekend. Many hospitals virtually shut down over the weekend, or at least they drastically cut back on their staffing and the related activities. Rehabilitative units, which operate in a much less intensive mode anyway, can become semi-dormant. But we were fortunate to have the weekend for Ruth to recover from the plane trip and the sedation. She was put in bed in a private room near the nurses' station so that the nurses could monitor her condition. She slept for almost forty-eight hours, though she awoke several times confused and distressed.

In rehabilitation hospitals and units expectations about time are different from what they are in acute care hospitals. Whereas an acute hospital measures its discharges in terms of a few days, rehabilitative stays tend to last several weeks. This more leisurely pace seems to extend to how much gets done in a day.

Rehabilitation is a covered benefit under Medicare. It is usually provided in designated rehabilitation units housed within general hospitals, though some rehabilitation centers may be entire hospitals themselves. The care in these facilities is distinct from the care often labeled rehabilitation that nursing facilities provide. The requirements of the latter are less stringent and the intensity of the rehabilitative care is correspondingly less. To be eligible for full rehabilitation, patients must be capable of improving their condition and must be able to tolerate at least three hours a day of active rehabilitation, such as physical therapy, occupational therapy, or speech therapy.

Ruth woke up briefly that first night and was out of control. Eventually we were called at Joan's home, where we were staying. We went to the rehabilitation hospital to try to calm her down but when we were not successful the staff felt it necessary to give her even more sedatives. In her agitated state she would slide out of the end of the bed if the bed rails were up. "Hospital policy," or the fear that she would fall and hurt herself, resulted in their using a form of a strait jacket, a soft cloth jacket restraint that kept her in the bed. She hated it. Although Robert had written articles about the dangers of restraints and the need to find other means to address agitated behaviors, his mother was now being sedated and physically restrained. Given the initial reluctance of the staff to even accept her as rehabilitation patients, however, he did not protest.

By this time, Robert realized that there is a huge gap between theory and practice. Although he knew the literature on the dangers of restraining people and hated the sight of my mother tied up, he had already acquiesced to such actions in the ICU because she needed IVs. Now we felt as though we had imposed on the rehabilitation staff.

Our mother was certainly not the ideal candidate for rehabilitation. Just managing her was proving an ordeal, especially for staff not accustomed to such patients. We felt guilty and impotent. We had no better plan to offer and wondered whether we had truly misled the staff about Ruth's rehabilitation potential. We tried to focus on simply getting through that weekend. Because we sensed that we were viewed as having misled the rehabilitation staff, we were reluctant to hang around, although we felt a great responsibility to see this episode through.

When Ruth woke up she was very confused. Some of her confusion was understandable. After all, she had been moved over two thousand miles without knowing what was happening. But when her confusion persisted, it was clear that her intellectual functioning had dramatically diminished. She did not know where she was even after we told her. Her short-term memory was poor. We will never know how much of her dementia was attributable to the stroke and how much reflected an underlying problem such as Alzheimer's disease. In essence, the etiology did not matter; none of it was reversible, although we learned with time that some of the symptoms could be made worse by medications. Although Ruth never regained her pre-stroke function, she did improve her cognition as some of the negative effects of treatment wore off.

Ruth vacillated between being agitated and being very docile. She had always had great respect for doctors (not that she followed their advice). Especially when they were male, she tried to please them. She might be a tiger for the female nurses to manage but she turned into a pussycat when the male doctor made rounds.

The rehabilitation process started slowly. The initial prognosis was very guarded. Ruth went to physical therapy, where they worked on building up her strength and occupational therapy that emphasized her coping skills. Because her slurred speech was hard to understand and she choked on some foods, she was evaluated by a speech therapist, who ordered a battery of tests, including a barium swallow to see whether her swallowing mechanism was intact. Fortunately it was, and gradually Ruth was allowed to eat more solid foods.

Initially she cooperated with the treatment regimen to the extent that seemed feasible, but after a week or so she became more resistant. As part of the rehabilitative process, the patients were encouraged to socialize and were expected to take their meals together. Even after she was well enough to participate in rehabilitation, Ruth would neither talk to nor eat with the rest of the patients. She just did not see herself as needing anyone but the staff and Joan, who was usually there to help her with her dinner. (After the first several days of rehabilitation Robert returned to Minneapolis, leaving Joan with the full burden of on-site care.)

Joan would arrive in the late afternoon after work to find Ruth in the hall in a wheelchair by the nurses' station because she could not be left alone in her room. Ruth's first reaction was always the expectation that Joan would "get her out" of there. At each visit Joan would have to spend a great of time talking to Ruth to get her to understand what had happened to her and that she could not function on her own. This ritual would continue through until the very end of this whole saga when Ruth just gave up and completely lost her will to live. The feistiness in her character most likely prolonged her life at the same time as it often worked against her.

Eventually, Ruth lost the luxury of a private room. Other patients' needs for privacy or care took precedence over Ruth's desire not to have to share her space. In the course of the next two weeks, two or three different patients shared a room with her. Each tried to find alternative arrangements. Sharing space, especially a bathroom, was always hard for Ruth, who valued her solitude. The additional fact that her sleep patterns were irregular and her mood swings and periods of agitation unpredictable only aggravated the situation for her and her unfortunate roommates.

The problem with roommates was the first of many situations in which Joan found herself in a somewhat conflicted state. Her loyalty and devotion were clearly directed toward our mother, but it was unpleasant to watch Ruth being rude and verbally or physically abusive to other patients, to some staff members, and even to Joan herself. Thus began another life lesson on this post-stroke journey: the need to separate one's own sense of embarrassment from the needs of the family member or other person for whom one is advocating. Not an easy dichotomy for Joan over the years.

Early on, Ruth became obsessed with getting to the bathroom if she had to urinate, and she seemed to have to go all the time. On several occasions she tried to get out of bed to go to the bathroom and fell. To keep a closer eye on her, the nurses moved her to a room nearer the nurses' station. The specific motivation to urinate so frequently was never clear. Ruth may have been suffering from a urinary tract infection. However, given her subsequent behavior, she may simply have developed a fixation with a constant need to urinate. A more thorough investigation of her incontinence was indicated but never conducted.

She had no patience and no ability to "wait her turn" for an aide. Many of the aides and nurses understood this as part of the post-stroke personality and tried very hard to meet her needs in a timely way, but some resented what they saw as a prima donna attitude. Unrealistic demands can create angry responses, but at the same time, one should not dismiss out of hand patients' expectations to have their needs met. The dilemma lies in establishing what is a realistic expectation and what is excessive. Ruth's emotional reactions and heavy demands were a central problem. She had good days and bad days, reminding us of the little girl with the curl in the middle of her forehead: when she was good she was very, very good but when she was bad . . .

Ruth gradually recovered her physical faculties over the next weeks. She could walk with a walker and then with a cane. Her cognitive function improved somewhat as well, and she began to reflect on her situation. For the first time since her stroke she said repeatedly that she wanted to die and blamed us for getting her into exactly the predicament she had feared most. She became visibly depressed and refused to cooperate with the rehabilitative regimen.

Robert tried to intervene by telephone. He called his mother to encourage her to participate actively in the rehabilitation. But the conversations were difficult. Her speech was still hard to understand and his entreaties were not persuasive.

Major schisms developed between Ruth and the staff. The floor nurses had great trouble managing her when she became agitated. They wanted to sedate her to make her more tractable. There were also concerns about her depression. Given the history in the ICU with psychoactive drugs, the physiatrist was reluctant to use such drugs. In desperation they called in a psychiatrist, who was expected to be skilled in the use of psychoactive medications, to initiate a drug program to raise Ruth's spirits, as well as to calm her down.

This psychiatrist was a remarkably caring, astute woman who took an instant interest in our mother and spent all of the Memorial Day weekend trying to get her in shape, mentally and physically, for the rehabilitation program. Although we had many conscientious and attentive medical personnel on our mother's case, this doctor was particularly special, not just because of her manner with Ruth but also because of the way she related to Joan, the lay member of the family. Joan always felt that this psychiatrist spoke to her as an intelligent person who could understand and process the medical terminology. Alas, this was not true of many other doctors whom Joan encountered in the course of the hospitalization and the next three years.

Considering the effects of the stroke itself and all the psychotropic medications that were administered, it is amazing that Ruth cooperated to the extent that she did. One problem that was never resolved was the conflict between Ruth's pattern of staying up late at night and sleeping late in the morning. In addition to dealing with the ramifications of her illness, the medical system was trying to make an owl into a lark. In the rehabilitation setting, this attempt to alter her diurnal rhythms was particularly difficult and frustrating for all concerned. Rehabilitative situations demand a great deal of compliance and cooperation, but all her life, Ruth had never been one to conform.

On the weekends, Joan spent as much time as possible visiting with our mother. There was only one short physical therapy session on Saturday morning and no therapy of any kind on Sunday. Fortunately, the weather was mild and pleasant during those first weeks, so the patients could be wheeled outdoors for fresh air and a change of scenery. On the weekend the mood on the floor was much more relaxed and patients were allowed to sleep later than usual. For Ruth, this was a good thing. She was still resisting the whole notion of being on anyone's timetable other than her own. Although she was incapacitated and sometimes confused, she still managed to reflect her old self. As frustrating as it might be, her obstinacy could be viewed as an indication of her autonomy.

Despite being on occasional sedatives, Ruth made remarkable progress. It is impossible to say how much of this gain was attributable to the rehabilitation and how much represented the natural course of her disease. Rehabilitation costs are paid for by Medicare on the condition that the patient make steady progress. Once a patient reaches a point where little further progress seems likely, the issue of discharge is raised. And when a patient is hard to manage, as was our mother, the incentive to discharge her is especially great.

The physiatrist, who had offered only a guarded prognosis, now announced that Ruth had reached her maximum and suggested that we begin to look for a suitable place to which to discharge her. "Once she can swallow and stand," he said, "she no longer needs to be here." Just as with the acute hospital, we suddenly felt Ruth was being propelled out the door. The suddenness of this decision to discharge her caught us by surprise. We had not made plans for the next step in her course.

We now found ourselves under pressure to find an appropriate home for our mother The discharge planner assigned to our case was a social worker in the rehabilitation facility. Her approach only made our task more difficult. She assumed that we had no real understanding of our mother's habits, likes, and needs—factors that are important parameters in finding a new living situation—and allowed us little time to give sufficient thought to what environment would be best for Ruth. Like most discharge planners who are employees of a hospital, her advice focused on what was expedient and available.

Now that the team had decided Ruth was ready for discharge, the leisurely rehabilitation pace picked up. The rehabilitation staff began emphasizing the need to find a suitable "placement," assuming that the next logical step was a nursing home. But Robert had spent much of his career studying the problems with quality of life and quality of care in nursing homes and was not about to put his mother in a nursing home until all other options were exhausted.

Although we spoke daily by telephone to discuss preferences and

options, most of the burden of finding a post-discharge location fell
to Joan because she was on the scene. The basic choices for Ruth at
this stage were going to a nursing home, moving in with Joan with
personal assistance, or moving into her own apartment with personal
care attendants. Joan's house was too small and poorly designed for a
person who had trouble walking, to say nothing of the interpersonal
dynamics that would make such an arrangement untenable. Ruth's
cognitive status was better but it was still not clear whether she could
function well on her own or supervise personal care attendants.

We believed that an appropriate place for a person with Ruth's
needs and social circumstances would be what has been termed "assisted living." In its original concept, assisted living implied a living
setting that provided at a minimum a private room and a bathroom
(or more typically a small apartment), modest food storage and preparation facilities, a door that could be locked, and a set of personal
care services tailored to one's needs. In assisted-living settings, the
notion is that people who previously might have needed a nursing
home could receive individually tailored care in their own quarters
while retaining familiar possessions and control over their life and
living space. Decisions such as when to go to bed and when to get up
are not made as part of an institutional routine. Assisted living was
premised on the view that needing assistance should not require giving up one's basic rights. It was designed to combine some aspects of
group living, such as meals in a communal dining area, and some ef-
ficiencies associated with round-the-clock staffing to oversee a group
of residents. In this sense it offered more security than home care in a
private home.

As the assisted-living concept gained momentum, however, it was
continually re-invented. Now almost every level of assistance can be
encompassed under that term. Moreover, different locales offer differ-

ent service packages called assisted living. For example, in New York, the range of care offered under this banner is much more restrictive than that offered under the same name in Oregon, where the modern concept emerged. Because of this range of definitions, we faced great frustration in seeking an assisted-living setting for Ruth.

We hoped to find something conveniently located near Joan that could provide an attractive living situation with competent staff. Unfortunately, there is no mechanism to facilitate such a search. The rehabilitation center's social worker made a few suggestions, but these were based on her limited direct experience. Little information was available about any of these places. It is ironic that one can now use a computer to look at hundreds of houses through a realtor but the service available to select a nursing home or an assisted-living facility is very primitive by comparison. It provides some information on the results of inspection but no real sense of the place.

We did what one usually does in such situations. We asked friends for recommendations. While Robert and his wife consulted with professionals, Joan used her own contact network. The professional route turned out to be very disappointing. Referrals to so-called experts produced only general comments with little specific data about the quality of facilities or commentaries on their features. By contrast, the informal network yielded lots of experiences. It is amazing how many people have family members who have used long-term care. It is a topic that no one talks about, although it features prominently in so many lives.

Assisted living was just beginning to develop on Long Island. Several facilities had been built or created from other buildings. Many were struggling to fill their beds. It turned out that most of the facilities were owned by the same small band of chains. Several places emerged with positive recommendations. Joan visited all of these to see firsthand what they looked like. But how do you really tell what a place is like? Most assisted-living facilities have a sales office. Although the sales people were friendly, we knew enough to approach them with the same caution one employs in a used-car lot. They have a product to sell. No assurances are too great, no claims too exaggerated. Because family, not the resident, is often the real customer, many assisted-living facilities invest heavily in the look and feel of the common areas. This is what people see when they come in. Little of it is ever used by the residents, however. For them the salient aspects are the rooms where they live, the food, and the staff.

We identified an assisted-living facility that had been created from a former motel. The rooms were sizable and each had its own bathroom. The food looked appetizing. Meals were served in a dining room that resembled a restaurant. The staff assured us that they were committed to providing good care and could handle our mother. In an effort to induce occupancy, they offered a large discount for the first six months from the monthly costs of about six thousand dollars. Like other facilities, they also required a substantial nonrefundable fee up front. A few moments' calculation showed that this introductory offer was highly attractive. We could try it out to see what our mother's life in this setting would be like without making so great a financial commitment that she would be stuck there. However, what the program correctly banks on is that inertia and the stress of finding another place will keep people in residence once they move in. We learned later that early "fill up" is an important goal for assisted-living firms because it allows them to attract more capital for expansion. Thus, deeply discounting six months' rent made economic sense for the firm.

The facility's location was also a major attraction. It was close to Joan's house and a few blocks from her husband's business. Although it may have been possible to find a better place somewhere else on Long Island or in the vicinity of New York City in terms of care, the difficulty for Joan to visit or to be available for emergencies would have been high. When we considered those factors, it seemed that Joan's ease of access offset any reservations we might have had about care. Having Joan nearby made a difference in both quality of care and quality of life.

The rehabilitation hospital planned Ruth's discharge for a Friday, but Joan was leaving that day for the wedding of one of Robert's daughters in Minnesota, and there was no one else who could facilitate the move for Ruth. In addition, Joan felt she needed to be nearby in case Ruth's initial adjustment to her new setting proved upsetting and difficult for her. We now found ourselves in the role of supplicants, asking the hospital to keep her for a final weekend. Joan promised to return Monday morning at eleven to transfer Ruth to the assisted-living facility we had chosen. Ruth was extremely agitated when Joan arrived Monday morning. She was clearly impatient to be out of there. During these periods of anger, frustration, and physical aggression, there was little Joan could do to please her. Then the moment would pass and Ruth would revert to being compliant, pleasant, and very grateful for all of the help and attention. This pattern continued right up until the end of her life and never got easier to deal with. Regardless of the different medications we tried, this behavior would occur any time Ruth felt stressed or abandoned. Such behavior, we found, creates mixed feelings in the caregiver. Guilt and anger merge. No matter how much you learn and understand about the brain and the effect of a stroke, it does not get easier to watch a loved one (or anyone) in this nasty, agitated state. One minute you feel angry and unappreciated and the next guilty that you are not doing more to prevent such outbursts.

Looking back on the rehabilitative experience, we feel that the treatment itself was a great success. It got our mother to the point where she could speak, eat, walk, and live a more normal but limited life. By the time of her discharge, she was speaking quite clearly, although there was some residual slurred speech. She was walking with a cane but tired easily. She had some episodes of incontinence but was able to use the toilet without assistance. She had short-term memory problems, but they did not seem to interfere with her daily functioning. She had a tremor that made eating messy.

Again, no one can say with certainty how much of her improvement was the direct result of the care provided and how much was the natural course of recovery. Probably those who were on duty when she arrived were quite surprised that she progressed as well she did. No doubt, there was a sigh of relief when she checked out as well.

LESSONS

1   Rehabilitation in a residential institution is not necessarily a seven-day-a-week process. The weekends in such facilities can be especially long for older patients.

2   Physiatrists vary in their knowledge of geriatrics. They may be uncomfortable handing the medical aspects of an older person's care or may fail to recognize when medical problems are adversely affecting recovery and tolerating rehabilitation.

3   A person's biorhythms are hard to change. Someone who has habitually slept late in the morning is not likely to adjust to the rigid schedule in an institution that starts the day early.

4   Formal rehabilitation provided in a designated rehabilitation unit must be distinguished from rehabilitative services provided in a nursing facility. The two types of care are paid for differently under Medicare. They require different levels of activity tolerance

by the patients and different clinical expectations by the clinicians. To be eligible for Medicare coverage a patient must be able to tolerate three hours a day of active rehabilitation.

5   Rehabilitation coverage under Medicare is time limited. Because Medicare pays for rehabilitation on a case basis but nursing homes are paid on a daily rate, the pressure for discharge from the former is heavy. The average stay in a rehabilitation unit is shorter than that in a nursing facility.

6   Family members can be helpful in the rehabilitative process. As with any hospitalization, their vigilance is a great safeguard against mistakes being made. But because family members have a natural instinct to be protective of their relative, they can also, in their concern, interfere with a process that requires a fair amount of pushing and prodding.

7   Rehabilitation units are now required to complete formal assessments on admission and at discharge to document the gains achieved. It is difficult, however, to separate the effects of rehabilitation from the natural course of the disease. There is some data for some conditions (such as stroke) that indicate the clear benefits of rehabilitation, but for others we are still trusting our instincts. Furthermore. the course can be different for different people.

8   Given a choice between using psychoactive medications and using behavioral therapy to address behavioral problems, most institutions unfortunately will choose the former, although there may be strong side effects.

9   Despite the slower pace of care, which should, ideally, provide time to make post-discharge plans, rehabilitative hospitals have the same incentive as acute hospitals to rush the discharge process and to stay removed from the clients' hard choices about where to go next. Families may need to take the initiative.

10   The process of discharge planning should involve consideration of two separate but related groups of questions: First, What type of care is best? Which is most likely to achieve the most important

treatment and care goals? What are those goals? (i.e., How does autonomy compare with safety?); second, once you have decided on the type of care, Which vendor is best suited? Here access and availability become central concerns, but so too do ambiance, quality, and life-style. Some places may have specific (or more subtle) policies about taking patients on Medicaid (or allowing people to stay once they convert to Medicaid).

11 Visiting potential discharge sites and considering what is involved in moving there is time consuming. It is easy to become impatient and grab the first open spot available.

12 Some potential options at discharge may be foreclosed because of the difficulty of arranging them. For example, it is easier to arrange a transfer to a nursing home than to work out all the details needed to initiate home care. Likewise, it is even more difficult to establish home care if the patient has no home to which she can return.

Assisted Living

When we brought our mother to the assisted-living facility in June 1999 she thought she was moving to a hotel. Her perception was quite apt, since the building had originally been a motel in a well-known chain. The new owners had created an attractive common space, with dining rooms that featured wait staff, recreational areas that included a theater with large-screen TV for showing videos, an all-purpose area with a small kitchen stocked with cookies and beverages for guests, and even a pool table at the entrance, which was much more likely to be used by visitors and staff than by residents. Much of the furnishings seemed to have been designed to attract families more than residents. The place was tastefully furnished and carefully decorated but the knickknacks were glued in place, perhaps a sign that the administration wanted a place that was homelike but not so much like home that you could actually enjoy anything, or risk harming it in the enjoying.

Ruth's room looked very much like what it had been originally, a fair-sized motel room. She had her own bathroom and a refrigerator, sink, and microwave oven that were arranged against a wall, hotel style. Closet space was minimal for a place of permanent residence. Her room had a small terrace that overlooked the grounds. Overall, Ruth seemed content with it. It was all the space she said she wanted. She liked the idea that she was in a hotel.

Although some people like to imagine assisted living as replacing nursing-home care, the range of services available at what we will call Terraceview were more suited to reasonably healthy older persons who had decided that the effort required to maintain their own households was too much but who were still quite capable of looking after themselves. A substantial number of the residents used canes or even walkers, but with these devices they could function independently. The emphasis was clearly on creature comforts rather than support. Great efforts were made to provide attractive and tasty meals. A recreational program ran all day with various group activities, including bus trips to a nearby mall several times a week.

The assisted-living facility went through the motions of performing a major assessment on Ruth to determine just how much assistance she would need and hence how much her stay would cost above the basic room-and-board charge. Because she had considerable disability from the stroke and was somewhat confused, they set a price that was supposed to cover substantial assistance from care staff (about six thousand dollars a month once we were paying the full rate). As things worked out, she received little hands-on help, though the staff was required to respond to the crises she created.

The basic package included cleaning the room and changing the linen weekly. Residents were expected to make their own beds, if possible, on other days and maintain their premises. Since our mother thought this was a hotel, she expected to have her bed made daily.

And since we were on an individualized plan that included our paying a higher rate than the base price because of the additional supervision she would require, we were eligible for the daily bed-making service. The Terraceview staff told us, however, that the bed could be made only in the mornings when housekeeping personnel were there. Ruth preferred to have her bed made later. With some effort we got them staff to agree to make her bed when she wanted. They considered this agreement a huge concession.

Most residents brought their own furniture, and the facility supplied linens. Having moved under emergency conditions from Florida, however, Ruth had no furniture. We rented some from the facility and bought some additional pieces, including a television and a stand for it, a comfortable chair and side tables, and some wall treatments.

Ruth also needed a new wardrobe. The dress of the day was basically loose elasticized exercise pants and tops, which were easy to put on and take off and, most important, washed well. Our fastidious mother, who fretted over her appearance, was now decked out in the most casual clothes. Moreover, the stroke had left her with enough residual weakness that her eating was messy. One glance at her clothes after a meal could reveal the entire menu. For the first few months after the stroke, Ruth was aware enough still to monitor her clothing and overall image, but gradually she grew unaware or indifferent to how she looked. Even when she was still interested in looking nice and being admired, however, she did not seem to notice the stains on her clothes, perhaps because of a combination of her failing eyesight and the effects of her stroke. But Joan was very conscious of our mother's messy appearance and was disturbed by the threat it posed to her dignity.

Ironically, despite the limited array of very simple outfits Ruth wore and her waning interest in her appearance, she still wanted many of her former clothes with her. One of her favorite activities was arranging the clothes in her small closet. In her former apartment every type of garment had its own storage device, and her wardrobe filled the closets in several rooms. Now she was restricted to one small closet. Fitting even her limited wardrobe into this space became a logistical challenge.

On days when she was feeling particularly well, she would want to wear a more special outfit. Some years earlier she had given Joan her fur coat. Now Ruth was delighted when Joan brought her to coat to wear on special occasions. She also had an elegant cape that she loved to wear when she went out.

Once it became clear that Ruth would never return to her Florida apartment, we had to undertake the task of closing it down. Robert and his wife were going to be in the area and agreed to pack up the belongings that she could keep with her in the assisted-living facility and close up the apartment. Going through the apartment, seeing how few of Ruth's once loved and carefully cared for possessions had any lasting meaning and recognizing that she had left her apartment in the midst of a stroke and would never return to it again made them profoundly sad. There had been no opportunity for any sort of closure.

Ruth had some fine pieces of furniture and was anxious that they go to her grandchildren. Unfortunately, the expense of shipping the furniture would have been far greater than its worth. It was never distributed. Robert and his wife boxed up Ruth's most portable possessions and shipped them off, leaving the rest to be sold when we put the condominium up for sale.

The experience of closing and selling the condominium revealed all of the irrationality that major life changes induce. Ruth had acquired a lot of possessions, mainly clothes but also furniture. She still had a ten-year-old car, which we sold to her mechanic. Once word got out that she was gone for good, various people came forward. The building janitor made it clear that he would like some of her possessions, and the man who had replaced our mother as the condominium president offered, for a modest fee, to oversee the sale of the condominium. Once we decided to leave most of her furniture and appliances there and to sell the condominium as it was, it seemed clear that it would likely become a carcass to be picked over. But trying to sell used furniture and appliances just did not seem to be worth it.

We had expected that Ruth would be terribly saddened at the thought of never again seeing the apartment she had worked so hard to furnish and perhaps feel that the dismantling represented a major point of decline in her life. To our surprise she seemed indifferent to the idea that her home was gone and to have accepted the idea that she was now permanently in New York. She did worry a great deal, however, about her jewelry. She believed that she had a large cache of valuable jewelry in her condominium. In truth, most of it was costume jewelry and the rest was generally of only modest value. But its sentimental value was very high; she wanted to distribute it among her daughter and granddaughters. She also wanted to have some of it with her. This desire raised a serious question about the overall safety of her possessions. Was it wise to leave even modestly valuable jewelry in the care of someone who was cognitively impaired? It seemed like a great temptation to the staff. In the end we left her costume jewelry with her but kept the few modestly expensive pieces at Joan's house and brought them in for special occasions.

Consistent with her basic lack of sociability and her compromised function after the stroke, Ruth chose to participate only in the dining component at Terraceview. She expected that Joan, who visited daily, would provide most of her entertainment and diversion. Joan would take her down to a late afternoon game or music activity; otherwise Ruth rarely left her room between meals, except when the staff came and spent time encouraging her to join an activity.

Terraceview also offered what they euphemistically called "wellness care," which meant a licensed practical nurse watched over the taking of medications and performed basic health checks, such as periodic weights. However, this was a very limited service. Ruth had developed congestive heart failure and would occasionally retain fluid. Robert attempted to organize a program of daily weights linked to a change in her diuretic medications to allow a timely response in the event of early signs of fluid build up, but the staff were unwilling to take even that much responsibility. It did not matter that we had arranged for a doctor's orders outlining the steps to be taken.

The first night in the facility was difficult. Ruth became agitated and disoriented. The Terraceview staff called Joan and asked her to come over to calm her mother. Ruth called Joan several times a night during those first few months when she had the ability to use the telephone and could remember the number she wanted to dial. To help Ruth, and to make it easy for therapists and aides who came in to reach her, Joan put a book near the bed with telephone numbers where she could be reached during the week and on weekends. At that point Ruth still had some concept of time. She could usually keep a fair track of the weekdays and weekends, but she could not be relied on to remember what she did in therapy or whether a therapist showed up or not. Often she would refuse the treatment, preferring to rest.

The early months of the stay in Terraceview featured few medical problems. In fact, Ruth used fewer services than those she was entitled to under Medicare. For example, Medicare covered in-home (or in this case, in the assisted-living facility) physical therapy services to help with her stroke recovery, but she was often not cooperative or compliant and eventually refused the services.

Her emotional adjustment, her very demanding way with the staff, and her refusal to get up and dressed in a timely way seemed to be the most controversial aspects of her care plan. A major issue with any form of institutional living is the extent to which the efficient operation of the facility should dictate the life-style of its residents.

Ruth went to the dining room for lunch and dinner but not breakfast. As far as we could remember, our mother had never gotten up for breakfast. Although the facility policy was that all residents should come to the dining room for all meals, Ruth's maintained her pattern of staying up late and sleeping late. She resisted getting up in time for breakfast and when she did get up, she wanted to eat in her room. Worried about her missing a meal, the staff generally acceded and brought her a tray. For the other meals she ate at a table for six. Assignments were fairly fixed, although people could petition to change their table. Indeed, our mother made just such a request. She was particularly unhappy at the first table placement after a man spoke rudely to his wife. She was already unhappy there because one of the other women was difficult and argumentative. Ruth never got along with women who were as assertive and forceful as she was.

Her new dining companions were a mixed lot. Most were more functional, certainly more cognitively intact than Ruth. One man. however, was actually more cognitively impaired. The women formed a fairly close group and seemed to support each other. Initially they seemed very kind to our mother, who could participate in the conversations, often taking her usual controversial stances. They seemed to tolerate her sloppy eating and even reminded her where things were or helped with ordering from the menu. But their tolerance did not last long. They began to complain to the staff and suggest to Joan that her mother really needed a part-time companion.

Private Aides

Although the term *assisted living* implies the merger of care with a comfortable living environment, we discovered that this was not the model we had bought into. Terraceview's expectation was that despite our paying for a basic set of services, we would hire outside help to look after our mother as it became necessary. The hiring of private duty aides was very prevalent in this particular setting (and indeed in the geographic area). Several residents had twenty-four-hour companions who were a common sight in the lobby or at the various activities. We often noticed tension between the regular staff and the aides over where the responsibility of one ended and the other began.

We started using outside aides part-time as companions in the afternoons to give Ruth more one-on-one attention. We hired people who were not certified aides but who were willing and able to devote a few hours a day three days a week to keep Ruth company. Then we added weekend aides, because it was helpful for Joan to have someone who could stop by for a few hours on the weekend so she would not have to keep coming in from her weekend home farther out on Long Island. Next it seemed a good idea to have someone to get Ruth dressed just before lunch and oversee the lunch hour. Although Ruth was usually a good eater, her appetite could become very poor when she was depressed or had an undiagnosed infection, and we thought that she would do better with a little one-on-one encouragement. By this time the other women at the second of her table placements were monitoring her eating and her behavior and they reported signs that she was not doing as well as she had been. These tablemates gave Joan reports on Ruth's food intake and overall mood, as well as any problems she was having with the dining room staff.

Joan found several people who were willing to work for the small amounts of time required to come in to get Ruth up and ready for lunch. These women would also stay with Ruth during the meal to encourage her to eat and to assist her a little. Our mother enjoyed the company and the attention, but then she began refusing to go to the dining room on some days. She preferred having the aide bring her meal back to her room, where the two ate alone.

One of the companions rarely showed up and another was doing the work more as an act of kindness than as a source of income. Hiring these women was not a long-term solution and created the additional problem that Ruth came to have a high expectation for one-on-one attention beyond what was needed to meet her immediate care needs. She wanted to be entertained or at least paid attention to even when there was nothing specific to be done for her. We discontinued this initial arrangement after the first of a series of hospitalizations and basically never reinstated it. On her return to Terraceview, Ruth always took a few days to readjust, then seemed to get back into the pattern of going to meals and eating regularly. In fact, sometimes she would order food, eat it, and then ask for something else, forgetting that she had eaten.

After each hospitalization her return to Terraceview was difficult for her. At one of these transitions hiring aides seemed an appropriate solution. In March 2000 Ruth was in the hospital for a fairly lengthy stay (almost a week), this time with pneumonia, and we realized that we would have to hire private aides to augment the care she would get when she returned to Terraceview. Her demands for assistance were too frequent to be met by the limited staff at Terraceview. She could not wait to be taken to the bathroom and she was becoming confused and agitated in the evenings, a phenomenon known as sundowning.

Early in her course we had hired aides for only a day or two to facilitate the transition back to Terraceview. After about a year we hired an aide to work as her full-time companion and assume much of the day-to-day responsibility for her. We were torn between wanting to meet Ruth's needs and demands for attention and our goal of preserving her functional independence. Taking this step undoubtedly made our mother more dependent. She needed the help, but more than that, she loved the attention. Hiring the aide also relieved Joan. She continued to visit Ruth almost every day but felt a sense of relief that the care burden was being met in part by someone else.

Even when Ruth had an aide during the day, the problems continued. When the aide left at 7:00 P.M. Ruth would panic. She started calling Joan after seven every night. Sometimes telephone reassurance sufficed but on numerous occasions Joan had to make an additional trip back to Terraceview to calm her down. For a while we hired both a daytime and a nighttime aide. However, when we realized that the night aide was doing nothing to control Ruth's wandering or her disruptive behaviors, we cut back to one twelve-hour daytime aide.

Ruth alternately fought with her daytime aide and basked in the pleasure of having someone to wait on her. In truth the aide was primarily a very expensive babysitter. And there was little for the nighttime aide to do other than watch Ruth sleep or roam around her room. Still, Ruth became dependent on having the aides. When there was a night aide, she liked the idea that the woman would fetch her breakfast before going off duty.

Initially we hired the aides through employment agencies, but the hourly rates were very high because of the inclusion of overhead and the agency fee. (We paid the agency about fifteen dollars an hour for aide services, of which the aide presumably received considerably less.) When it became clear that we would need a permanent night aide, we decided to hire someone directly. We could pay twelve dollars an hour and both parties would be better off. In the end one of the agency workers took the job.

As Ruth's condition deteriorated, the facility put pressure on us to have an aide during the night as well, despite our previous experience. Ruth was wandering around the facility at night, often spending time at the front desk. On several occasions when the staff tried to persuade her to go back to her room, she became very upset and once she was physically violent. At other times she knocked on the doors of other residents, prompting complaints.

A critical issue about Ruth's behavior at night was determining what could be expected of regular staff. The Terraceview staff seemed to feel nobody should be up and out of his or her apartment or room at night and did not think that it was their job to visit with people at night or attend to them. Moreover, the layout of the facility made it difficult for the smaller night staff to attend to the residents. Although assisted-living rates are considerably lower than those of a nursing home, when the cost of hiring aides is included, the two become much more comparable. In fact, the cost of adding a night aide as well as a day aide would mean that Ruth's care at Terraceview would be more expensive than the care offered in a nursing home. We pointed out that we were already making extra payments for incontinence care.

The facility staff said that our providing twenty-four-hour aide care was the only condition under which they could allow Ruth to stay. The conflict over the use of aides and Ruth's increasingly agitated and problematic nighttime behavior eventually led to our moving her.

Indeed, many families hired full-time aides, or at least full assistance while the older person was awake. As we spent time with the aides we had hired, we found that there was a whole community of aides in the facility who worked together and knew each other. We were not the only family required to supplement the meager services Terraceview provided.

Even with the presence of an aide during the day, Ruth still slept until nine or ten most mornings and participated only rarely in activities. The aide we hired directly, Phyllis, was fond of playing bingo, however, and would bring Ruth along to participate passively. Gradually her behavior seemed to improve and we gave up the night aide. Phyllis would come in for a ten-hour shift, which allowed her to attend to all of Ruth's grooming needs and see her through meals. Indeed, under Phyllis's care, Ruth looked much more presentable, a fact that Joan appreciated greatly. Her clothes were almost always clean and occasionally she even wore make-up. She looked more like her former self.

Phyllis seemed to understand Ruth. She came almost every day for many months. She was positive and upbeat and she learned quickly how to handle Ruth, getting her to do things better than most other people could. She was usually able to flatter and cajole Ruth out of her bouts of anger and seemed to know when to leave the room and give her a chance to cool off. We valued her devotion, her reliability, and her warmth. Phyllis was very sociable; it was important for Ruth to be stimulated and part of the group, even if she chose not to be. The rationale for employing Phyllis was that she was prolonging and improving the quality of Ruth's life, but in many respects Joan's life was benefiting at least as much. Joan felt she could make shorter visits to Ruth, knowing she was in good hands and that she had someone who would advocate for her and keep her safe in Joan's absence.

Ironically, Phyllis's loyalty and sense of duty to our mother brought her into conflict with the facility. Although Terraceview had insisted that we hire someone, the staff did not appreciate her making demands for services our mother was entitled to or pointing out when purchased care was not provided. On our behalf she was monitoring the care actually provided by the facility and they did not appreciate it.

In an assisted-living situation it is not always easy to know when more help is needed. One of our reasons for having the aide was to stimulate Ruth to join in activities. It seemed better that she be out of her room most of the day. Another benefit was that with someone to look after her appearance Ruth was much cleaner and neater. Finally, she was more sociable in Phyllis's company; she talked more to the other residents and aides in the lobby and enjoyed watching other people play pool and socialize.

On good days Ruth entertained others with tales of her past exploits and conquests. She liked to talk about people she had met and romances she had had. She tended to exaggerate in describing herself as an adventurer who had regularly defied social convention and led a glamorous life. Her favorite stories were about the relationships she had had with men after her husband's death, especially with the man fifteen years younger than she and the son of one of her neighbors in Florida who used to sneak up to her apartment during his visits to his mother.

We began to wonder whether all this added attention from Phyllis was worth the added expense. Joan would arrive almost daily to find

Ruth dozing while Phyllis was nearby playing Bingo, an activity that broke up her day and the monotony of her job. Yet Joan was comforted to know that when she was not there Ruth was not alone. This was the greatest irony of all—that this supremely independent woman who had kept to herself most of her life past fifty-five now hated to be alone. She would become frightened and disoriented after seven o'clock when Phyllis left, exhibiting the behavior that prompted us to begin hiring nighttime aides.

Perhaps the situation was exacerbated by Ruth's getting so much attention during the day and then having none at night. It is hard to determine how much of the anxiety was induced by Phyllis's leaving in the evening and how much was the result of a natural progression and manifestation of her type of dementia. Ruth's relations with her aide ran hot and cold. She had tirades during the day and several times evicted her from her room. After each episode she would be contrite, reverting back to a sweet, compliant, almost child-like personality. It was a very difficult pattern to watch and follow.

Her behavior was reminiscent of what it had been in years past. Ruth had always had a bad temper and was prone to making stinging statements in moments of anger, but she was also flirtatious and coy. She could assume a pose and charm people. Now she seemed to be doing it in a more docile way. It was as if the shadow of her stronger earlier self was following familiar patterns but with less potency. She had often been described as a "tough cookie" with strong opinions and an acerbic tongue. She considered herself an excellent judge of character, and when she detected what she called a "phony" would not hesitate to point it out. The old Ruth, who had often given rides to hitchhikers, tended to root for the underdog and was usually sensitive to people in the service community. When Ruth's personality seemed to change after the stroke, it was hard for Joan to watch. She felt sad and embarrassed. She never got used to witnessing Ruth's rudeness or her out-of-control behavior. Ruth would make comments about people's appearance or actions without any inhibition.

Medical Management

In the fall of 1999 Ruth experienced the first of what was to become a series of hospitalizations for congestive heart failure. The Terraceview nursing staff (who were not registered nurses) would understandably get very nervous when she said she could not breathe. It was difficult for untrained staff to distinguish between shortness of breath as a sign of anxiety and real shortness of breath due to heart or lung disease. They were unwilling to take any chances. Because they were unsure about why Ruth was short of breath, she was sent to the hospital.

Each of these congestive failure episodes followed the same pattern. At first Ruth would receive large doses of diuretics, which created a constant need to urinate. Patients in the hospital's emergency room (ER) with congestive failure were not allowed to go the bathroom on their own, but at the same time the ER staff could not or would not facilitate frequent trips to the bathroom. Instead they preferred to catheterize Ruth, and then she would be admitted to her hospital room with the catheter. It always became an issue and a struggle to get the catheter removed because she was such a handful without it, especially with all of the diuretics she was getting. Finally, the doctor would write an order that the catheter be removed; but it could take up to half a day for this to happen, depending on the situation on the ward. Ruth would now be getting weaker and more atrophied from lack of walking or whatever limited ambulation she had been used to. She would become weaker, barely eating, and then would eventually be discharged in a far worse state than when she arrived with the congestive heart failure.

Ruth seemed to vacillate between retaining excessive fluid and becoming dehydrated. Either condition could set off a series of adverse events that affected her both physically and mentally. Robert attempted to work with the so-called wellness staff to have them monitor her situation more closely. He explained that dehydration was a serious problem with substantial potential consequences. When he asked them to remind her to take fluids regularly, they said that reminding her to drink water and orange juice was not allowed in their license. They construed that simple act as delivering health care. They were there to provide her with food and drinks but not to take responsibility for her intake.

As this terrible cyclical pattern became familiar, we tried desperately to break it. Ruth's first doctor was quite understanding and actively tried to avoid keeping her in the hospital, but sometimes the wheels were set in motion without his consent or knowledge. Not only did each hospitalization provoke a physical setback, but Ruth's return to Terraceview after each hospitalization became more and more difficult for her.

As noted earlier, at one of these transitions hiring aides seemed to be a good solution, though taking this step undoubtedly made Ruth more dependent. In addition to constant aide care, Joan still continued to visit her almost every day.

Not every hospitalization provoked a crisis. Ruth complained of stomach pain one day and was taken to see her geriatrician, who diagnosed an umbilical hernia. He recommended a surgeon, who agreed to do the corrective surgical procedure (basically pushing back the protruding part of the intestine and securing the weakness in her abdominal wall) as same-day outpatient surgery. Ruth was a real trooper for the surgery. She tolerated it much better than she had the care for other ailments, perhaps because by that time she had a full-time aide to stay with her upon her return to Terraceview. Another factor could have been that she was in and out of the hospital in one day and did not have a chance to develop the patterns that set her back with each stay in a hospital.

When she first moved to Terraceview, Ruth could walk with a cane (and sometimes without one). She moved slowly but she was ambulatory, and we would walk around the facility and the grounds. We would take short trips to go out for lunch or dinner, and Joan would take her to the beauty parlor. Ruth continued to use only a cane until December 1999. By that time she was weaker or less motivated to walk by herself; and several people suggested that she use a walker.

Like every aspect of our mother's life after the stroke, her behavior became unpredictable and each day was a new experience. She could go through a fairly smooth period for a few weeks and then a new crisis would arise, causing us to question whether we were acting in her best interests. Any change in her health seemed to affect her mood and her behavior. Her appetite and her overall energy level would decrease. The medical staff were slow to make this connection, if indeed they ever really did. In retrospect, it now seems that many of her major behavioral changes were linked to bodily infections that often went undiagnosed until they were acute.

Indeed, atypical presentation of illness is one of the hallmarks of geriatric medical practice. Most of the manifestations of illness, or what we call symptoms, are not so much the direct effects of the illness as the body's reaction to the stress of an illness. With aging, the ability of the body to respond to stressful situations decreases.

Thus, if older persons lose their capacity to respond, it follows that the manifestations of their illnesses will be more subtle and will not necessarily correspond to the typical presentations of these problems. In older people, new disease events do not announce themselves as vividly as they do in younger people. Pneumonia in an older person, for example, may present as confusion or fatigue. Even a heart attack can present this way. Clinicians and those caring for older persons need to be alert for subtle changes in behavior, which may represent important changes in health status.

Likewise, one form of illness may precipitate other problems. For example, when Ruth's congestive heart failure got worse or she developed pneumonia, her mental status might deteriorate, leading to behavioral outbursts. If these new episodes reflected a change in her physical health, psychoactive medications might not be the most appropriate treatment.

Coordinating Ruth's medical care presented a problem. She needed a primary care doctor, and though a few doctors made regular visits to the facility, their credentials were weak. When Robert looked them up in the directory of medical specialists, he found that none had training in geriatrics, and so he called his geriatric colleagues in the area to look for a referral. A geriatrician in the same geographic area as her earlier rehabilitation hospital came highly recommended. When Robert called him, he was already heavily scheduled but agreed to take Ruth on as a patient. He was very obliging but this arrangement posed several logistical problems. In addition to the time required for the visit, and for waiting, the trip to the doctor's office took thirty minutes each way. It was challenging to work all that into Joan's schedule, because she taught elementary school every day. Moreover, the geriatrician did not have attending privileges at the hospital closest to

Terraceview. That meant that an emergency admission could lead to a hospitalization where Ruth's primary care doctor could not take care of her.

Infections were a problem too. Ruth often developed urinary tract infections or an upper respiratory infections that would go undetected until she stopped eating, became weak, or appeared clearly to be in a much worse than normal state. Although we were paying for the top level of care, the Terraceview staff were generally remiss about noting this syndrome. Upper respiratory infections continued to be a problem for which she was treated (but not quickly enough) many times in the last three years of her life. In many instances these infections were associated with changes in her behavior, suggesting that physical problems could exacerbate her cognitive state.

Deterioration

Ruth's physical and mental health gradually declined. She had increasing trouble walking. With assistance from the facility and a prescription from her doctor, we ordered a walker. Right before our eyes our mother was turning into a frail older person. It was frightening to watch.

Efforts to get her interested in outings and activities other than doing laundry in her sink and rearranging her closet, tasks that harkened back to her former life, generally failed. She was always meticulous about doing the laundry and she loved her clothes. When she first went to Terraceview she had insisted on washing her own underwear (and hanging it on the terrace to dry). Part of the motivation was probably a desire to hide the incontinence she had developed, but part, too, was falling back on lifelong behaviors. Unfortunately, not only did she create a Neapolitan tableau for the neighbors but she could not get the laundry clean. Joan would take the items home and rewash them with the rest of Ruth's clothes.

Ruth did enjoy going out for a meal or a visit to the beauty shop. It gave her a chance to dress up a bit. She could wear some of her more elegant clothes, especially a cape that gave her a sense of panache. Unfortunately, every meal outing meant a big dry cleaning bill.

As her mental state deteriorated Ruth began to wander at night, a problem that was intensified when she started knocking on other residents' doors in the middle of the night. She would roam the halls in search of snacks or water, often half naked. Ruth had lost the ability to monitor her behavior and seemed not to realize how inappropriate it had become. The problem was exacerbated by the way she would lash out in this state of anxiety, using verbal and physical abuse against all in her path. Afterward, she could show some remorse for what she had done, but generally she appeared not to remember any of these antisocial behaviors. One night she left the faucets running after doing her washing and flooded her room. Her inability to remember any of these misadventures was extremely frustrating. Indeed, she would vehemently deny them

About a year into her stay at Terraceview, her troublesome behavior necessitated our bringing in a psychiatrist at the behest of the Terraceview staff. We chose one who already worked with the facility in the hope that he could help the staff develop a coping approach that would minimize the use of psychoactive drugs. The staff, however, needed reassurance that Ruth would be sedated enough to avert the disruptive adventures. We thus began a perilous journey to find the right combination of medications that could control Ruth's behavior without prompting somnolence or an adverse reaction. There is no predetermined level of drug for these purposes. Finding the right dosage is best accomplished by observing the patient closely for a time and making a series of minor adjustments. Unfortunately, the Ter-raceview staff was not up to the task. Even with prompting, they were unable to organize any systematic record of observations that could enlighten the prescribing physician. Instead, the psychiatrist's actions were based largely on responses to crises. Alas, there was no shortage of those.

As the situation deteriorated, the facility called us in for a case conference and insisted that Ruth have an aide with her every night. After failing to convince them that there were other ways to solve the problem, we agreed to hire someone. We could appreciate that they were short-staffed, especially at night, and that Ruth required more at-tention than they could provide, but hiring a full-time attendant who could assist only our mother seemed very wasteful and extravagant. We suggested that there were likely other residents with similar needs (as indeed there were) and that it made economic sense for each fam-ily to pay a little more to buy, in effect, part of a person's time who could then oversee several clients. The facility, however, did not want to become involved in any such arrangement that would require their taking responsibility or initiative. Their solution was to require each family to hire its own aides. Basically the facility told us that either we would have to hire a night aide or be prepared to move our mother to their "dementia" unit, where staff was said to be more accessible dur-ing the night.

It became quite clear by that summer of 2000 that she was going to have to be moved either within the facility or to a new facility. Her memory loss combined with the effects of the stroke made it impos-sible for her to remember directions—even those that involved her safety. The final blow occurred when she was found on the terrace after dinner one night and her hand was badly cut. We had asked staff to lock her terrace door, but they would not, so she continued to go outside in the evenings alone. The cut on her hand required yet another trip to an ER. The problem was made worse because she needed her hand for balance and this meant it would take longer for the wound to heal properly. Again, each minor injury or even short-term visit to an ER or hospital stay had a more long-term deleterious effect on our mother.

Ultimately her behavior worsened. She wandered more, and her eating got sloppier. She would go out to the front desk or call them to demand help. The facility reached its limit of tolerance; staff claimed, probably truthfully, that the other residents were complaining about her. They presented an ultimatum: either move her to another facility or transfer her to the special care unit (SCU) that Terraceview operated for persons with dementia. Without alerting us, they had actually put her in the SCU in the middle of the night when she had flooded her room, much to the distress of Joan, who came the next day to visit and found that Ruth had been moved downstairs. We knew then that she could not stay at Terraceview.

The Terraceview dementia unit was effectively a locked ward in the basement. Though the rooms were comparable in size and layout, much of the charm of the décor in the upstairs rooms was lacking. In truth, it was ugly, and life there was much more regimented. This clientele ate separately from the rest of the facility and rarely left the unit. We had fought hard against the idea of a nursing home, but now our options were rapidly diminishing. At one point when Ruth's behavior became very severe, the geriatrician had suggested that she would likely need to enter a nursing home. He recommended one that had the best reputation in the area for dementia care. Thinking we had few other options, we went to see it. Although it was well staffed with a full-time geriatric psychiatrist (probably the reason it had such a good reputation), it was a bleak place. There were few single rooms.

The rooms were devoid of furnishings. The regimen was strict. The other inmates (indeed, that is the best word to describe them) could provide little company. If this was the kind of care our mother needed, it meant giving up the last vestiges of quality of life. Now we had to evaluate our options. We were determined to search for something else that could provide basic care in a less dreary environment.

As a teacher, Joan had a frame of reference different from that of the medical profession, but she could readily see parallels. The placements and decisions for special needs students are always based on the "least restrictive" environment. We wanted much the same thing for our mother: the most normal situation possible. What is best for the patient is often not pleasant for the other members of that community. This social conflict was becoming apparent. However, once you put someone on a "dementia" unit, the equivalent of a "self-contained special education placement," his or her behavior can decline rapidly for any number of reasons. Expectations are lowered and the behaviors the person observes in others makes him or her uncomfortable. When we eventually did move our mother to a special dementia unit in a different assisted-living setting, as the next chapter describes, she regularly complained about the crazy and inappropriate people all around her. She was sensitive to noise and commotion, so it was a real problem that one of the women wandered around moaning or screaming much of the time. Fortunately, however, in all of Ruth's moves she never had to share her room. Sharing space was troublesome under the best of circumstances for our mother.

Once we accepted the idea that we would have to move Ruth into a different unit, we started to think about whether a more major move was in order. Since we were no longer pleased with the attention and care Terraceview was providing and did not like the ambiance of the dementia unit, a more complete move seemed reasonable. Moreover, we were still uncomfortable with the idea that our mother had to be in the special dementia unit with all of its restrictions. We visited several assisted-living facilities, including a new one that was just opening in the same general area, hoping to find a more tolerant environment that provided a higher level of care than Terraceview did. By this time we had learned to be skeptical shoppers. We met with the administrator of the new facility to discuss the feasibility of transferring Ruth. She was very reassuring about their commitment and capability, insisting that they could handle a wide range of problems. For every dilemma we posed she had an answer. But she really had no concrete plans for how to manage someone like our mother. Indeed, she was not a health professional but a salesperson, and it was pretty clear that her enthusiasm was largely a reflection of her strong desire to fill empty beds. We quickly learned that empty beds can produce empty promises.

LESSONS

1 The term *assisted living* has come to mean anything a vendor wants it to. It is used to describe board-and-care homes with shared rooms and few amenities, housing with services programs built around various levels of housing and meal plans, and programs that combine proactive services with life in a very comfortable, very livable environment. The original concept of assisted living was based on the idea that it is possible to offer a reasonable living situation and the services a person needs. The setting featured enough living space that a person could control, including a bedroom, a private bathroom, and at least minimal resources to store food and prepare simple meals. Today it is not uncommon for a service described as assisted living to be provided in shared space not any better than that found in nursing

homes. In general, you get what you pay for, but the formula is never that simple.

2   You have to be very careful to understand just what a facility that describes its service as assisted living is prepared to do. It is important to discuss specifics and be skeptical of general assurances. Even then, the promises made on enrollment may not be kept. The more you can get in writing, the stronger your position will be.

3   The people who discuss living in the assisted-living facility are often not the ones who run it but salespeople working on commission. The reassurances they offer may prove to be baseless.

4   You may have worked with an engaging salesperson in the initial stages who assured you that all your needs can be met. Salespeople, however, have little influence, if any, on how a resident is handled once the contract is signed.

5   Your position is never strong. Even with full disclosure, residents and families are at a great disadvantage in negotiating with assisted-living staff. If the staff claims they cannot manage a resident, what does the family gain by proving them wrong? What is the value in forcing a facility to keep a resident they feel inadequate to manage? In the end they can always fall back on incompetence. You can complain loud and long and even threaten to sue, but what will you achieve? What is the point on insisting that the facility do what it says it cannot? In the end, you do not want to insist on getting care a facility says it cannot provide.

6   The following issues should be clarified and put in writing before a decision is made:

•   What services (and how often and to what extent) will be provided as part of the fee? Usually there is a base package and often several increments above that. Some places are very flexible about what is included and others are not.

- How can additional care be purchased (i.e., increments and cost)? Will the facility provide it or must it be obtained independently (see lesson 11 below)?
- Do they have the capacity to provide more intensive personal services? How are these services priced (usually in fifteen- or thirty-minute increments)?
- What other charges are involved (e.g., community-service fee)?
- What is the facility's expectation about your having to hire outside help? What is their commitment to provide care when you do?
- What is the staffing ratio?
- What arrangements have been made for nursing oversight, if needed (e.g., dispensing medications, checking blood pressure or weight)?
- What is the relationship with sources of medical care? Who is on staff to carry out physicians' orders? How is the communication with the client's physician managed?
- How many meals are provided? How are they priced? Are they charged whether eaten or not?
- What are the policies about individual life-style choices (e.g., when to get up or go to bed, missing meals)?
- What are the criteria for admission and, especially, discharge? How disabled can a person become and still remain a resident?
- What types of problem would indicate that the assisted-living facility cannot care for the client (e.g., severe behavioral problems, aggressive or disruptive behavior, incontinence, needing a wheelchair, level of medical problems)? The criteria for admitting someone may be more restrictive than those for retaining them. Many facilities are willing to take care of people who, in effect, age in place.

7   Assisted living is not the same in all states. Most states have some statewide information, which can be obtained through the federal Administration on Aging (see Appendix 2).

8   Assisted-living facilities generally cannot and should not care for the full spectrum of frail older people found in nursing homes. The challenge is to identify which portion of that spectrum they are well suited for. Many assisted-living facilities prefer to restrict their care to people who really do not need much assistance. Others seek to provide care on a par with that of nursing homes. Some of this difference is driven by state regulations. Some reflects the market niche the assisted-living facility is aiming for.

9   Assisted-living facilities will continue to look to family members to intervene in crises and to provide services.

10   The assisted-living facility's assurances that it can handle any situation may be predicated on your hiring a nurse's aide or the equivalent. This service will be an added cost and may not reduce the fees you are paying to the facility. The combined costs may easily exceed what you would pay for care in a nursing home, but one of the advantages to such an arrangement is that the person is living in a much nicer situation.

11   Unfortunately, even when families are willing to purchase extra care, there is no easy way to organize it to ensure that you get the amount of extra care you really need. As a result you may end up having to hire a nurse's aide full time when you really need such a person only part time. Assisted-living facilities could make this extra staffing work better for everyone if they organized a staffing pool that allowed cooperative purchasing of extra aide time. Some facilities will sell additional care incrementally, usually in fifteen-minute intervals, but that time is not always dedicated and accountable.

12   Assisted-living facilities should provide for flexible staffing that can be affordable on an additional hourly rate by creating the equivalent of the "permanent sub" concept in a school. For example, one or two staff members would be in attendance daily to cover

emergencies, provide one-on-one care, and allow for additional coverage if a resident's condition worsened. They could even be used to accompany patients to the emergency room.

13   Assisted living should make it possible for families to buy additional staff on an hourly basis. While families may not want to enter into a new negotiation each time a modest amount of additional effort is needed, when substantial additional supervision or assistance is required, it should not necessitate hiring outside staff who must work full shifts for one client. Some system that makes the additional care more affordable and better integrated would be preferable.

14   Make sure you see the actual room promised, not just the common space or some showroom.

15   In older people, cognitive and even behavioral problems frequently are set off by physical changes. For that reason, it is very important for staff to be alert to subtle changes in a person's status. Family members, too, need to think about the possibility that the behavioral changes that are frustrating and upsetting them might be subtle reflections of some underlying medical exacerbation. Unfortunately, many doctors are not familiar with how disease presents in older persons and may not recognize what is happening. They may even reject these suggestions from family members.

16   Most assisted-living facilities do not view themselves as health care providers and are very likely to respond to a resident's health problems by sending the person to the emergency room.

17   Primary medical care for assisted-living residents needs to be more closely coordinated with the care given by the assisted-living facility staff. The staff needs a close working relationship with the doctor. Too often patients are sent to emergency rooms because communication with physicians is poor or doctors are unwilling to see residents in the assisted-living facility. Perhaps greater use of nurse practitioners could alleviate some of these

problems. The nurse practitioners could help to educate staff and make the necessary "house calls."

18   Assisted-living facility staff members are rarely trained to get actively involved in tracking medical conditions and reporting any changes in a resident's status.

19   Most assisted-living facilities are fearful about external regulators. They are risk averse, avoiding any situation that leaves them vulnerable to criticism or legal action. They will not undertake any task that may get them into potential difficulty. Hence, they are reluctant to do anything creative or to tailor programs to individual needs.

20   Problem solvers are rare. It is hard to get staff members to think creatively about how to mange a behavior problem or even to be willing to use solutions that a resident's family might devise. The combination of fear of regulations and lack of creativity is a major stumbling block to developing effective care.

21   Personnel change can be a problem. Staff members who seem more helpful and sympathetic than others may suddenly be transferred, for example, to a new facility to train other people.

22   Many older persons do not share personal space easily. They do not want to confront frailty if they can avoid it. Thus, because of fears and frustrations, residents are not always kind to each other, especially in situations where frail people and those who are noisy and aggressive are housed among those who are more intact.

6

The Dementia Unit

About the same time that it became clear that we would have to make a major relocation decision, Joan decided to move farther out on Long Island, where she would no longer be at a convenient distance from Terraceview. Close to Joan's new home, however, was an assisted-living facility operated by one of the largest national chains, whose president had championed the ability to serve complex cases. The complexity in Ruth's case lay in her behavioral outbursts and the need to manage her medical conditions, which could exacerbate her mental condition. Beyond that she needed a supervised environment, although her mental status was still amazingly sharp in many areas.

Robert's wife had met this company's president at several assisted-living conferences and he had spoken proudly about how his facilities were prepared to take on even the most difficult cases. She offered to call him to assess the ability of the facility to manage a case as complex as Ruth's. He responded positively to the challenge and assured us that they were up to the task.

It happened that we were together in New York, along with Robert's wife, a few weeks later, and to take advantage of our VIP status, we arranged to visit the new facility, which we will call Sunset. We met with the administrator, who had obviously been briefed. We tried to describe our mother's behavior as frankly as possible. The administrator was encouraging but at the same time cautious. She cited her long experience and appreciation for the kind of assistance people with dementia need and said that their "reminiscence unit" would be best suited for our mother. This euphemism described a locked, albeit well-appointed, area with special staffing. Each resident had his or her own small studio apartment with a full bathroom. The overall unit was organized with the dining and living areas and the galley kitchen as the focal point. The large living room and smaller sitting rooms were stocked with costumes and other memorabilia of earlier times. The unit boasted a pleasant patio where residents could get fresh air, but a protective railing kept the residents in. Several cats lived in the unit. Altogether it was a pleasant spot. The ward was basically locked. The elevators, which were the main means of entering or leaving, required a pass code designed to be inoperable by the residents. Several residents always seemed to be stationed by the elevators trying to get downstairs, though they never seemed highly motivated to leave.

Because the administrator expressed some uncertainty about whether they could handle a resident like Ruth, despite the national program's frequent claims that it could manage complex cases, we negotiated a sixty-day trial. In effect, Ruth would be there "on approval." The administrator proposed a modification of their usual contract. Like many assisted-living facilities, they levied an additional, so-called community service fee, which was supposed to cover the cost of communal amenities. Whatever it purportedly covered, it was actually an extra payment equivalent to the first three months' fees, over and above the monthly charges, that seemed to us to be no more than a device to cover the upfront costs should a person decide to leave after only a few months. For us, this fee would be pro-rated and then applied to Ruth's account if she stayed.

With some trepidation, given the modest commitment of the Sunset staff, we made the move. The new facility was close to Joan. The parent company had a better reputation than Terraceview.

In addition to the physical relocation, we also had to arrange for new medical care. Robert called the nearby university medical center and was able to get one of the geriatric care faculty to agree to take her on. Since this geriatrician worked closely with a nurse practitioner (NP) who made regular rounds every two or three weeks at Sunset, much of the care could be done on site. We hoped that the regular presence of the NP would lead to closer coordination of the care with the Sunset staff. This goal was only partially met. The NP was accessible but still could not respond to the emergency needs Ruth experienced. Also, we elected to use a psychiatrist who was already affiliated with Sunset and came well recommended in the hope that he could coordinate closely with the staff. We were especially pleased because he seemed to want to avoid psychoactive medications as much as possible. All of Ruth's now extensive medical records were copied and transferred.

The period immediately after the move was traumatic. Ruth never liked the new location. She hated being with "crazy people." Indeed, for much of the time she outwardly appeared to be much more normal than most of her fellow residents. She could converse coherently as long as no memory was required. She managed to charm many of the staff, who adopted her as their pet resident.

Although she had not objected to the idea of moving from Terrace-view, her dislike for her new accommodations was evident. Geron-tologists allude to "transfer trauma," the stress of relocation, although its extent is still debated. Some of Ruth's reaction may have been due to the move itself, but much of it was prompted by the fact that this was a dementia unit. Ruth did not see herself as someone who needed to be around demented people. She insisted that Joan could care for her in her new home. She proposed living by herself in an apartment. When we countered that she could not live alone, she suggested that we hire someone to stay with her around the clock. She had no insight into how hard it would be to sustain help for her. No efforts to rea-son with her would suffice. The repeated discussions were especially frustrating. Much of what we were doing was reiterating the same arguments because she was unable to recall what we had just ex-plained. Her insistence that she could function independently in the face of such obvious incapacity was more than ironic; it was draining. It was hard to retain our composure as we went through the same script again and again. To our further frustration, she was using the telephone in her room to call random numbers, another indication that her cognitive functioning was diminishing. When people started complaining about these "crazy calls," we had to take the telephone out of the room.

Perhaps responding to her frustration, she became very restless at night. In contrast to the reaction at Terraceview, the Sunset staff suggested that Joan stay away for a few days to give Ruth a chance to adjust. This "take charge" attitude seemed encouraging. During the probationary period Robert was in regular telephone contact with the administrator, and everyone seemed committed to making this placement work. The prominence of Ruth's son and daughter-in-law in the geriatric health care field was clearly a factor in motivating the staff to try to make things work.

Certain times of day seemed to be more difficult for Ruth. Lunch hour was particularly bad. Whether it was the result of the diuretics starting to work or just her diurnal clock, she seemed to be more agitated at noon. Often she would actually overturn tables in her rage and several times she threw tableware. Joan had to buy a set of plastic dishes and cups for her use in the dining room. Early on in her stay, the staff tried a variety of behavioral approaches to reduce her agitation. The aides bathed her in the hot tub to help calm her down, but the bathing seemed to bring on frequent urinary infections that would cause a loss of appetite, exhaustion, and weight loss. Joan even bought tapes of Frank Sinatra, whose singing Ruth had always enjoyed, and mellow music to try to calm her moods. None of these efforts seemed to help consistently.

Her evening tirades became more active. Somehow this frail little old lady was able to destroy her room. The staff responded by removing everything breakable. The room now resembled a monastic cell. As the behavioral approaches failed, they turned to the consultant psychiatrist, who put her on small amounts of medication. He was anxious to avoid overdosing. While the medications seemed to help with her night fits, they made her very drowsy. She was now tractable but very sleepy.

Despite a continuous habit of wandering at night and periodic outbursts, which included trashing her room, Ruth did eventually pass her probationary period. By this time the psychiatrist had become actively involved and the staff felt they could manage her with a combination of medications and attention. Perhaps because of pressure from above, the staff was committed to working out a plan for her. They negotiated a rate that was considerably higher than what we had paid at Terraceview ($6,700 a month). This rate was supposed to cover the added staff attention and incontinence care. None of it was covered by Medicare.

Not surprisingly, Ruth rarely interacted with any of the other residents. She ate by herself at a separate table. Her sitting alone turned out to be a good thing because she would often throw glasses or dishes when agitated or frustrated. At Terraceview she had developed a fixation about needing to go to the bathroom constantly, and this behavior continued at the new facility. No sooner would she sit down than she would insist that she needed to use the bathroom, though often it was possible to distract and redirect her. She was able to sustain a conversation, usually based largely on reminiscing or discussing her family. Indeed, one could use the same conversation over and over again. If she became engrossed in these talks, she would forget about her bathroom fixation. Joan and Robert used these ploys frequently, and the staff did as well when they paid attention. The level of attention varied greatly with the staff member on duty.

Ruth's cognitive function was extremely spotty and inconsistent. She might repeatedly ask where she was and forget what she had eaten ten minutes before, then surprise us by making a remark that reflected a high level of irony. For example, one day when Robert and his wife were sitting with Ruth on the facility's veranda a cat came by. Ruth had no love for pets in general and especially not cats. Robert remarked on the cat and Ruth said she didn't know where it came from. He explained that it belonged to the facility and, as such, it belonged in part to her. She immediately responded, "You can have my share." Another time we referred to some roses we had brought the day before. Although they were out of sight in her room, she remembered them accurately. When we asked her why she could recall them, she said "I remember what I like." However, about the same time she had no recollection of a visit from one of her grandsons, of whom she was very fond.

This era in our mother's life was not without some almost pleasant moments. During a lovely celebration the unit put on for Valentine's Day, Ruth, who loved the music and the attention from some of the male workers, actually stood up and danced in place to the music and a photograph was taken. That picture captured a lighter, happier moment in a very sad and frustrating chapter of her life. The staff often reminded us during the declining months that followed about how animated and contented she had seemed on that evening.

During the first six months, when Ruth's nighttime wandering was becoming a greater problem, Sunset was stressed. Experienced staff was recruited away from Sunset to start two new facilities the company had opened in the same general region. The administrator who had committed the staff to working with our mother was among the first to leave. Several staff followed. Moreover, the supervisor of the dementia unit went out on maternity leave. The remaining staff was both short-handed and less experienced.

We soon discovered that Sunset's boast about being able to handle difficult cases was conditioned on the premise that families hire and pay for their own, supplemental staff. The facility strongly suggested that we hire a private duty aide to oversee our mother at night, to prevent her wandering the corridors and knocking on other people's doors. Although we were presumably paying a higher rate for "dementia care," they had no provision for our simply paying a little more for more oversight. They wanted us to hire someone from the private agency that was licensed to come into their facility, but they did not want to get involved in making the arrangements. We were expected to contact the agency on our own. This demand seemed inconsistent with the image the national chain was trying to create of being able to respond to care needs. We learned, however, that our experience is common in assisted living, where the extent of the assistance is quite limited and families are expected to hire their own help, at an additional cost.

Recruiting aides, even through agencies, was never easy. In the early days, when we were hiring day-by-day, availability was always a problem. As we moved to more permanent arrangements, reliability became an issue. Promised help did not always show up. Although the facility staff had pressed us to hire the help, they took no responsibility to notify us when an aide failed to show up.

The night aides were frustrated with Ruth's behavior and lack of sleep. She could be very abusive as well. In the course of about a year, she went through no less than twenty different aides. In addition, we found ourselves responsible for paying for care that was not given. The aides would show up later than the arranged 11:00 P.M. start time and leave long before 7:00 in the morning. The facility staff took no responsibility for monitoring their attendance. We were often not told about the shorter hours until Joan had already paid the full bill in good faith. The private night aides were supposed to get our mother up, showered, and ready for breakfast, but they usually left before she woke up. The facility staff resented the private night aides' leaving before Ruth was up and ready for the day. On one hand, in all fairness, her erratic sleep pattern did not help. She was up so late at night that it was virtually impossible to get her roused before the aide was scheduled to leave. On the other hand, the role of the extra aide should not be to relieve the day staff of their work. Sunset had not reduced its rates to recognize any decrease in expected staff effort. Quite the contrary, in addition to providing our aide coverage, we were paying a high rate for assisted-living services. The issue of whose responsibility it was to get Ruth ready for the day caused friction between the private aides and the Sunset staff. This conflict together with our mother's wild outbursts made her a very difficult patient to manage. We had several conferences with the administrator and staff director to discuss these issues but achieved no ready resolution. They likely felt that it would be better if she left. Our relationship with the firm's president, however, made that option less viable.

Once again the issue of infections and their effect on her behavior and overall demeanor plagued Ruth. An exacerbation in her medical condition could worsen her behavior, and her behavior could make it hard to detect a change in her medical condition. She could be suffering with some low-grade infection that manifested itself by decreased appetite or more agitated behavior. No one seemed to make the connection between such an infection and its deleterious, yet subtle effect on Ruth. By the time anyone realized she was ill, what had begun as a cold was already full blown pneumonia and sometimes required hospitalization

Ruth's medical condition necessitated multiple hospital admissions. Periodically she would develop a chest infection that seemed to exacerbate her congestive heart failure. As before, she seemed to come back from each hospitalization in a much worse state than when she had left. In the hospital she became confused and agitated. Even the day trips to the emergency room proved draining and disorienting for her. One time when Joan arrived as Ruth was returning from an emergency room visit necessitated by yet another fall, she found her totally exhausted and furious at the same time.

The edema (i.e., swelling) in her legs was a major problem. Ruth began to develop sores on her legs that required many trips to the doctor's office, which was actually at a clinic in the hospital. At one point, Joan was taking her there two or three times a week. The Sunset staff was very cooperative about the follow-up care, but Ruth was often noncompliant and extremely averse to all of the bandaging. It was made more difficult because Ruth could not understand what was happening to her. She could not remember that she could not walk unassisted and would get up out of bed and fall yet again. The staff even moved her mattress to the floor so the falls would be less severe. Her room resembled a prison cell, except that there was a window and a television, which she never used. Actually the only people who watched the television were the night aides. Although Ruth used to watch television a great deal before her stroke, she lost interest in it right after the stroke.

Ruth's balance became worse with time. It is hard to say how much of the problem was due to the psychoactive medications she was receiving to control her behavioral outbursts and how much to her overall weakness, her poor eyesight, and her impatience. The facility became concerned with each fall. Although she had bad bruising, there was no indication of a fracture on any occasion. Nonetheless, to protect themselves, they wanted to call 911 each time she fell and have her sent to the local emergency room to be checked out. Not only did this action entail enormous expense for Medicare, but each trip created a major disorienting disruption in her life. We were able finally to convince the facility that we would sign a risk negotiation agreement, taking full responsibility for the consequences of these falls. Because we would much prefer to have Ruth active and falling than restrained and going to the emergency room, under such an agreement we would absolve the facility of any liability associated with a fall. Despite our offering to make such a signed statement, the Sunset staff was still reluctant. They felt at risk from citations by state inspectors as well as from any claims of negligence from us. Even though we were prepared to acknowledge that her continued activity would inevitably lead to her falling more, it was distressing to see her all bruised. If a social worker were to wander, in we were sure we would be accused of elder abuse.

What's more, not every fall could be handled under the risk agreement. One day Ruth fell and hurt the eye that had some years earlier been treated for a cataract with a lens implant. She was rushed to the emergency room, where an ophthalmologist was summoned. He stitched her cornea and admitted her for observation. Joan tried to call Robert, who was attending a national gerontology meeting, and left a message that was garbled into a suggestion that his mother "had poked her eye out." After several telephone calls it became clear to him that she had dislodged her lens implant. Fearing that she could lose what sight she had left, he headed immediately for the hospital.

When we visited our mother the next day at the hospital, a Sunday, we were impressed with the close attention she was receiving from the nursing staff. They stopped in regularly to check on her and sometimes just to chat. When Robert came back the next day, a Monday, the situation was totally different. The unit was a buzz of activity. Ruth, who was simply recovering, was the lowest priority. The nursing staff ignored her. Requests for assistance went unheeded. At one point Robert had to take her to the bathroom. Although she did not seem to mind when he half carried her to the toilet and oversaw her activity, he felt very embarrassed. In the absence of hospital staff, he virtually became her nurse's aide, helping her to eat and to dress, as well as make frequent trips to the toilet.

The situation with emergency hospital care was similar to what we faced in the first assisted-living setting. The hospital most likely to be used in an emergency was not one where her primary care physician had admitting privileges. Her primary care team admitted patients to the university hospital, but that was not the closest hospital. Thus, if an ambulance was called, the EMTs (emergency medical technicians) would take Ruth to the local community hospital where her primary care team did not have privileges. Her psychiatrist, however, did.

Not all of Ruth's hospitalizations were emergencies, and on one occasion at least, using someone other than her primary care team had a positive result. At one stage, the psychiatrist had so much difficulty adjusting her medications that he decided it would be best to admit her to the hospital where she could be watched closely as he reduced and then increased her dosage. He arranged to admit Ruth to the psychiatric ward of the local hospital. There it became evident that she was suffering from severe pneumonia, and she was transferred to a medical floor for treatment. Because her regular medical team could not take care of her there, an internist with no credentials in geriatrics was assigned her case. He discontinued her psychoactive medications and began to treat her medical problems aggressively. To everyone's great surprise, not only did she rally medically but her behavior became much more tractable. She was discharged back to Sunset with no psychoactive medications.

In the hospital, she was kept in a geri-chair by the nurse's station most of the day. A geri-chair is essentially a high chair for adults with an unmovable bar; it is classified as a physical restraint. Joan would arrive every night to help her with dinner. At some point in this episode Ruth lost her bottom dentures. Most likely she took them out in the hospital and left them on the tray when it was collected.

It was clear that Ruth was deteriorating both mentally and physically. Joan sensed it, but Robert could see it on his periodic visits. As a geriatrician, he knew that some of the problems could be iatrogenic, that is, caused by the treatments she was receiving; but he also recognized that her disease was progressing. However much he wanted to keep his mother out of nursing home, she could see that her need for care was becoming more than assisted living could provide, even with the supplementation we were paying for.

As her physical strength began to wane, Ruth experienced increasing difficulty ambulating on her own. This difficulty was complicated by the Parkinsonian side effects of the psychoactive medications, which had been reinstituted. At one point she became very rigid and could barely walk because of these side effects. Even with her walker she could go only short distances. She required a great deal of assistance getting in and out of a car, and. every trip became an ordeal. Although an athletic person, Joan often did not have the physical strength to manage all the steps needed in accomplishing a transfer in and out of her car single handedly. Robert feared that Joan was simply becoming timid and facilitating Ruth's dependency, and so to show her the art of the possible he proposed that they take Ruth out for lunch on his next visit to town.

When Robert came next we went to visit Ruth with Joan's husband. Robert believed that surely with three of us, we could manage an outing. We decided to take her out for pizza, which she enjoyed and could still eat on her own. Despite her stiffness, we were able to get her into a wheelchair and roll her to the front door, where the car awaited. With a lot of maneuvering, we got her into the backseat of the station wagon. We drove the few blocks to the restaurant and prepared to transfer her from the car to the wheelchair. Despite our best efforts, Ruth could not make the transfer. Indeed, she was so stiff she could not step up onto the curb. At one point with her son-in-law behind her and Robert in front trying to help Ruth into the wheelchair, she collapsed and fell backward onto the car seat on top of her son-in-law. It was so pathetic it was funny. All three of us burst out laughing. We loaded the ungainly mess of mother-in-law lying atop her companion in the back seat and drove back to the assisted-living facility, where we brought in the pizza. In the face of these severe Parkinsonian side effects, the psychiatrist discontinued the antipsychotic medication. The whole farcical episode pointed to a great truth. Members of the larger family caregiving team who see less of the patient than the one person providing care daily may feel the need to introduce a new spirit of activation to push the daily caregiver out of despondent routines, but sometimes their ideas can be naïve and unrealistic.

That was the last outing we attempted on our own. Any subsequent transportation required hiring a special van that could accommodate a wheelchair. Sadly, the next time Ruth traveled by car would be to enter a nursing home.

LESSONS

1   Assisted-living facilities are often designed more to attract families than to help residents. Their elegant architectural flourishes give the impression of nice hotels, but these attributes do not necessarily translate into better care. They may have gimmicks, such as a reminiscence room in the dementia unit designed to provide residents with an environment that invites them to revisit their childhood, but few residents ever actually use them. Studies have shown that families are initially seduced by these trappings of care but find that once the resident has been there a while they are of little consequence. In the end, the relationships between the caregivers and the resident prove to be the most important element of care. It comes as no surprise that caring is the most important aspect of caring. Unfortunately these relationships can be undermined when staff turn over.

2   Assurances that a facility can handle difficult cases need full disclosure. Do these assurances come with the assumption that the

family will hire private aides? In such a circumstance, you may be paying a high price for basic, insufficient care.

3   Assisted living is not a parking place for older persons, especially those with cognitive problems. Continued family advocacy and involvement is essential.

4   Staff turnover is common. What you see when you sign up may not be what you get later. If you make a decision about entering a facility based on the quality of the staff on duty then, be aware that many of them may leave within a few years.

5   Persons with some cognitive problems, especially with active behavioral manifestations, are not tolerated by the more cognitively intact. Nor do those with fewer cognitive losses necessarily do well in special units among severely demented people.

6   Nurse practitioners can be a useful form of primary care for institutionalized older persons if they are well integrated into the basic care system, empowered to act, and able to communicate quickly and effectively with primary care doctors.

7   Sending frail older persons to the hospital after every misadventure can take a heavy toll. Each admission can be disorienting and require a prolonged recovery period.

8   Hospitals do not attend well to the needs of frail older patients, especially once the immediate medical crisis has abated.

9   In an assisted-living facility, even well-intentioned staff may not be good problem solvers. Those who tend to focus only on responding to the immediate issues may not be willing to look for deeper underlying causes or to consider strategies that are not directly related to the immediate task at hand.

10 Managing behaviorally aggressive confused older persons in a calm competent manner is challenging, exhausting, and frustrating

11 Faced with behavioral problems, staff may too readily appeal for using psychoactive drugs.

12   Psychoactive drugs have potentially powerful side effects and often do more harm than good. They should be used with great caution and stopped as soon as possible.

13   Behavioral problems in confused older persons may be the manifestations of physical problems. Very often a worsening of a physical problem may set off a series of behavioral manifestations. It is therefore important to pay close attention to dementia patients' physical health status and to consider physical problems as the basis for changes in mental state.

Nursing Home

Sunset had made it very evident that they could no longer care for our mother. Hiring a full-time aide on top of the money we were paying for the assisted living that provided ever less assistance seemed unworkable and expensive. At the same time Ruth's financial resources were beginning to diminish rapidly. For the first time, we began to seriously think of her as a potential Medicaid candidate. If she were eventually to go on Medicaid we knew our chances of finding a good nursing home would be much improved if she entered as private-pay patient. Most nursing homes will give priority to patients who can pay with private funds and thus avoid some of the government oversight. Many of those private-pay residents, however, will eventually spend down to become eligible for Medicaid. Paying privately usually means higher rates but presumably somewhat better care and often nicer rooms.

With great reluctance, we set about to identify a nursing home for Ruth. This step, clearly a last resort, was especially painful because a career of studying long-term care had convinced Robert that nursing homes are socially (but alas not physically) sterile environments. Furthermore, our mother's only experience with a nursing home was the one she had had with her own father, who was so unhappy after he was placed in a nursing home that he tried to kill himself. That event left a scar on our mother's soul, as well as a profoundly strong reason to avoid such a placement for Ruth.

We found one nursing home in the area that came with very positive reviews from both the informal experience of family members who had used it and the official statistics available on the Medicare Web site that lists the characteristics of every nursing home and the results of the most recent federal survey (see Appendix 2). However, to be sure we were making the best decision, we arranged to visit several others.

Earlier we had visited the home recommended by a geriatrician as the ideal place to manage dementia. Although it had a full-time gero-psychiatrist in residence and a good complement of staff, it was a socially sterile environment that seemed to be heavily custodial. Moreover, it had few single rooms.

We identified several others by reputation and reviewed their characteristics on the Web site. When we visited each of them we were disappointed. The corridors were crowded with wheelchairs filled with people lined up for meals or baths or other activities. The residents looked uncared for, and the staff seemed to focus on avoiding accidents rather than enhancing the lives of the residents. Each place, even those newly constructed, seemed terribly institutional.

The highly recommended facility, which we will call Sincerecare, was part of a large campus operated by a nonprofit organization. Because we were told that there was a long waiting lists to get in, we decided to play all our cards. Robert called the medical director, who was familiar with his work, and explained our situation. He agreed to give us a personal tour. This facility, like the others, was institutional but here we got the impression of a great many staff and active efforts to make the place as hospitable as possible. These extras were affordable because of private donations over and above the fees charged. Indeed, the walls were covered with plaques acknowledging donors.

The facility seemed very clean and well maintained. However, even the newest addition was built with primarily double rooms. When we asked why, the medical director cited cost concerns. Many nursing homes that evidence great concern about their care, we learned, persist in building semi-private accommodations rather than single rooms. The often repeated concern that the cost of construction is prohibitive is simply not true. Moreover, the flexibility gained by providing more single rooms will help keep occupancy high.

Sincerecare had a fully staffed medical clinic on the premises that included several geriatricians who provided the primary care for residents. Even specialists came to the facility at scheduled times to see referral cases. Of all the facilities we had visited this was clearly the best, but even so it was not ideal. It was still a hospital-like arrangement with nurses in nursing stations and long bleak corridors. We felt we needed to make the best of a bad situation and pressed for information about availability.

We were referred to the admissions office and soon realized that we had been naïve about how long-term care works in New York. When we said that we expected to have our mother admitted as a private-pay resident, the admissions person was surprised but delighted. The fees for private payment (about $300 a day) were about twice what the state allowed under Medicaid ($186 a day), although the care provided did not seem to differ in any obvious respect. (It is important to note that these fees included the cost of physician care.)

Although the vast majority of their rooms were semi-private, we suggested strongly that Ruth would be much better off in a single room. Her behavioral problems superimposed on a long history of not sharing space well made her a poor candidate for a roommate.

We were given a large set of forms to fill out, some of which requested diagnostic information, but most of which were financial declarations. A caseworker was dispatched to complete a state-mandated evaluation to establish our mother's level of eligibility for nursing home care. The requirements for nursing home admission are much more stringent than those for assisted living, largely because the former are eligible for coverage under Medicaid.

We had been trying to manage our mother's funds prudently, but the costs of assisted living and the private aide plus her medications added up each month. Her expenses were outstripping the income she received from her investments and each month we were dipping into her capital. (Her money supply was hemorrhaging not dwindling, at this point.) It was clear that before long she would use up her savings and have to go on Medicaid. Several people suggested that we consult with an attorney who specialized in Medicaid financial planning.

This consultation proved informative. Although there is formally a requirement that the applicant have no assets for a period of three years, or at least that the state can attach any assets transferred during that time, in practice the state of New York has a certain formula that allows a person to pay for many months of care and then become eligible for Medicaid. The lawyer made some calculations and advised us to disperse the rest of Ruth's estate less enough funds to cover seventeen months. Since Joan already had power of attorney and was a co-signator on all Ruth's financial documents, this disbursement was not difficult to accomplish. In effect, we had begun to implement Ruth's will before her death.

A room in Sincerecare became available much faster than we had expected. Although it was a double, we were told a transfer could be made to a private room when one became available. We never knew whether this speedy admission was related to the fact that we were paying privately, but we were impressed that the room became available thirty minutes after the lawyer's letter of intention arrived at the Sincerecare financial office.

Although it seemed to be made as a "now or never" offer, Joan (with Robert's blessing) actually turned down the first room offered because it meant that Ruth would have to go that day and no advance warning or preparations had been made for the transfer. It was going to be a huge psychological leap from assisted living to nursing home for all concerned. Joan feared that Ruth would be extremely confused and disoriented. She was not in the middle of a health crisis and would not understand even in a limited way why a change was taking place. (One of the terrible side effects of the stroke was that Ruth, like many people with stroke, had lost the ability to understand why certain things were happening to her. It is also likely that this inability to process was the root of much of her anxiety.) Joan made the decision to wait for the next available room to give both Ruth and herself the weekend to try to adjust to the coming change. In retrospect, the wait proved to be a good decision because the next available room was a single. Joan and her husband drove Ruth to the new facility in their car. The Sunset staff were helpful and enormously relieved that the burden of caring for our mother was ending.

Ruth was neither pleased nor upset at the move initially. She liked the fact that there were lots of staff who gave her attention. She did not like the other residents, many of whom were severely cognitively impaired, but she had not liked living with her cohabitants at Sunset either. Because she had so little memory, she rarely made such comparisons. We were very careful not to use the words *nursing home* and at first she thought she was in a hospital. Because she was not in any medical crisis, it was a little hard for her to process why the move had taken place. But when she saw a plant that had been left behind by the former occupant of her room, she asked very specifically what had happened to him. Had he died? When we acknowledged that indeed he had died, she gradually seemed to realize this was not the kind of "hospital" she was used to, and after just a few days in the new facility she volunteered the idea to Joan that she was in a nursing home.

Sincerecare was a large, widely spread out facility with more than five hundred beds distributed over several units. Getting from one place to the next always seemed to require a long walk through a maze of corridors. The units were large, with a nurses' station at the convergence of three hallways. The dining room was large, and all the residents seemed to be fed at the same time. The facility had a formal way to doing most things. For example, all visitors were required to sign in and receive special visitor identity badges. When we checked Ruth in we brought along her television set on its rolling stand. The guard at the door told us to leave the set there. A maintenance person would bring it up and install it. Along the way they decided that the stand was not necessary and that the set could be placed on her bureau. Space was in short supply even in a single room.

Despite the obvious efforts to decorate the place and to make it seem inhabitable, Sincerecare was clearly primarily a health care institution. Social amenities were an afterthought if they were thought of at all. For example, there were no provisions to facilitate calling in on the telephone. To speak with Robert, Ruth had to be wheeled to the nurses' station and handed the telephone there, which had a short cord. No cordless telephones were available.

At the same time, much attention had been given to creating

various activities for the residents. On Ruth's bulletin board a weekly calendar of activities was posted, and early in her stay we noted that a current events discussion was being held and suggested that she might like to attend. Joan wheeled her down to what looked like a small gymnasium where an activities person was lining up her audience. Because each attendee had to be brought down by either family or a staff member, it took over half an hour just to gather the participants. The first step in the already delayed process was to take attendance. If Ruth was mildly interested at the initial idea, she lost interest by the time the activity got under way.

A large number of people were assembled theater style in a room with no furniture or appointments, just empty space and a podium. The activity leader used the podium very distant from the group rather than standing in the middle with a hand mike. A few people participated in discussing the hockey dad who had committed murder in Boston. Ruth, who had fallen asleep, suddenly woke up and said loudly "Help me," the phrase she used frequently to announce distress. Realizing that this activity was not working for her and that she was a disruption to the few participants who seemed engaged, Joan wheeled her out. The whole arrangement, Joan concluded, was a travesty. None of the participants had chosen the activity and if taking attendance were really necessary, it could have been done more efficiently. Indeed, large group activities attended by heterogeneous collections of residents are poor substitutes for meaningful activity. Real activities need to be tailored to the interests and tolerance of the audience, and they need to engage the residents more actively.

Ruth's vision, as well as her intellect, had deteriorated. She did not see herself as one of "them" (the other residents) in the sense that she had no idea of her own limitations and condition. This inability to see herself accurately was also a protective device. She would have suffered great distress if she had known how sloppy and unkempt she often looked. Appearances were still important to her and she scrutinized everyone with whom she came in contact.

The routine in Sincerecare was much more medical than it had been at Sunset. In addition to getting a complete physical examination, Ruth received evaluations from several members of the staff, including a physical therapist who devised an exercise regimen intended to get her walking again. In fact, she never got out of her wheelchair except for the designated exercise periods. When she would be taken down for physical therapy, she would often become frightened and disoriented and worried about how she would get "home." This anxiety would often prevent her from accomplishing the exercises and she would become noncompliant. Eventually, she stopped going to physical therapy because it was too upsetting for her. The aides would try to have her "walk" with support on both sides, but then, too, she would complain bitterly and refuse to take another step.

Because she had several episodes of choking, the nursing home ordered a barium swallow examination. Even though the results were normal, they put her on a soft diet and thickened all of her liquids to avoid aspiration. Essentially all food and beverages were almost the same consistency. Given her propensity to choke, she needed substantial assistance and supervision in eating. Because she did not react well to tablemates, she was seated at a table by herself. She hated the fact that she could never have a real liquid drink after that. She was constantly thirsty and yet she never felt her thirst could be quenched. She also despised the food.

The routine at Sincerecare was to serve her breakfast in her room, which was more in keeping with her diurnal clock and waking patterns. Recognizing her distress at not having her dentures, the staff also ordered the in-house dentist to make her a new set of lower dentures. The process took many visits and fittings. At times, Ruth would be transported down to the clinic and be so disoriented that the necessary work could not be performed. By the time the dentures were made, they were never comfortable in her mouth. Most likely, her weight had decreased enough to make the fit loose and annoying for her. She ended up rarely wearing her new teeth, but not for lack of effort by the dental staff.

Although she had formerly used a combination of a walker and wheelchair in Sunset, she now spent all her time in a wheelchair or in bed. The staff kept her up for most of the day. They required her to come to all meals and did not tolerate her sleeping late, although they did allow her to eat her breakfast in her room at the appropriate time.

She was taken off all psychoactive medications and appeared calm. The nursing staff was very attentive. Because they did not want her in a room alone where she could not be observed, she became part of a group of residents seated in front of the nursing station. Just across from the station was an open area with a television set that played movies and programs. About a dozen wheelchairs were always lined up in front of this set with people staring vacantly at it, including our mother, who had long ago seemed to lose all interest in television.

She looked as out of it as anyone, yet when someone went to her and roused her she would respond. Indeed, she was still capable of recognizing relatively unfamiliar people, such as her daughter-in-law, who came to visit Ruth alone and unexpectedly a few months before her death. Even people who are as severely cognitively impaired as Ruth was can interact, but it takes intensive individual efforts. Keeping people by the nursing station is supposed to help with that interaction, but it does so only if someone makes the effort to talk to them.

Ruth simply sat in her chair apparently lost in thought, but perhaps just lost. When we asked her what she thought about, she was vague, explaining that the time seemed to pass quickly enough even with not much to do. She still had the behavioral pattern of moaning and crying out her mantra, "Help me, help me," but was less able to articulate what she wanted help with. This cry was like a verbal tic with which she got revved up for sentences as in, "Help me, help me, how are you?" Eventually, because she would doze off frequently and her head would droop down, a reclining geri-chair replaced the regular wheelchair. The staff attached an alarm system that would go off if she got out of the chair and attempted to walk; she never did.

Joan visited her almost every day. Visiting seemed to be the norm at Sincerecare. The halls were always filled with family members wheeling their loved ones or just sitting and talking. The expected level of active family attention was so strong that much to our surprise, when Joan had a period of planned absence for a week's vacation, the facility suggested that we think about hiring someone to come in to keep our mother company. The facility's social worker offered this visiting service. It seemed outrageous to us that at the rate we were paying for care, they would see an extra hello from activities persons or social workers while Joan was away to be such a big deal. In fact, Robert came in to fill up many of the missing days. One of the auxiliary volunteers made a habit of stopping by to see our mother. She would spend some time sitting with her and trying to engage her in conversation. Even though her contacts were infrequent, Joan was very grateful that someone was taking the time to give our mother some personal attention.

Because Joan visited so often and because engaging Ruth in conversation was so difficult, she kept her visits short. By contrast, Robert came much less frequently, but his visits tended to be longer. Irrationally Joan felt guilty because her brother stayed so long. Somehow she felt the difference in the lengths of their visits reflected poorly on her commitment to her mother.

On one occasion we both visited Ruth with our spouses and decided to oblige her in her desire to play bridge. Ruth had regularly lamented the lack of bridge partners at all the places she had been. Despite the fact that she had no short-term memory and had lost most of her vision, she persisted in seeing herself capable of playing bridge. We worked hard to keep the game going, playing her hands for her and consulting her about each action. But she enjoyed it and waned to play more hands. She seemed to like getting out of the nursing station area into the adjacent sunroom area and certainly enjoyed the personal attention from her family. Indeed she could be engaged but at what price? Few facilities can afford the staff to cater to each resident's individual whims and desires. More active use of volunteers might help to some degree, but it would take a large cadre of dedicated volunteers to meet the demand. Such burdens inevitably fall on families. Those residents without active family support are multiply bereft.

The family visits were difficult. It was harder and harder to maintain a conversation. Even the usual reminiscences were shorter. And with her appetite decreasing, we could no longer engage her by bringing in ice cream or Chinese food, once her favorites. In effect, she was disappearing before our eyes. Each day the traces of the person we had loved were harder to see. She had become simply a little old lady. Sincerecare was a very well maintained institution, but it was still an institution. It had a variety of rules and worked off a medical model. Residents were treated as patients who had problems that needed to be addressed, and this care was given in a structured environment. The nurses were extremely kind. They quickly established a bond with our mother and, indeed, seemed to know her as a person, but there was a clear hierarchy. The registered nurses delegated most of the actual care to the aides.

Ruth had both a primary care geriatrician and a psychiatrist to manage her medical needs. In contrast to her earlier care, they coordinated their efforts well. And, in contrast to her experience at both assisted-living facilities, which had sent her regularly to the hospital, during her entire stay at Sincerecare, despite her deteriorating condition, she was never transferred to the hospital..

After all her assessments were completed, the staff held a case conference to develop a care plan. Joan was invited to the conference, but, to her frustration, it was scheduled in the middle of her teaching day, and despite the Sincerecare staff's assurances that they wanted Joan's active participation, they made no effort to reschedule. Joan did attend, but the assigned social worker was not present. A substitute social worker attended in her place, making Joan's special effort seem futile. This important meeting could well have been rescheduled for the convenience of both Joan and the social worker, two key participants. At the meeting a formal plan of care, including rehabilitation, was laid out. Emphasis was placed on keeping Ruth safe, including altering her diet to accommodate her dental problems. A new set of advance directives was created, which, actually, was simply a recapitulation of her previous ones.

Ruth had moments, even hours, of relative calm and lucidity. She still had a sharp wit if she were initiating the jokes or witticisms. For a time her legs and body were very swollen with edema, causing her to look heavier than her actual weight. So when Joan came back after five days without seeing our mother, she was shocked to see the dramatic changes that had taken place. Ruth was tiny and much thinner than she had been. She was much weaker overall and barely responsive.

The head nurse even noticed that this was the first time that Joan's arrival did not elicit the big smile and happy reaction that normally occurred, clearly a sign that Ruth was giving up and going inside herself even more. Joan asked the nurse whether her mother was going to die soon. To her credit, the nurse was frank but kind and let Joan know that a lack of response like this was often a sign of a further and serious decline. At every visit after that, which, it turned out, was two weeks before Ruth died, it seemed as though Ruth was just slowly wasting away in front of her daughter.

Ever since the stroke Ruth had experienced periods of agitation and moments when she would lash out at the person who was there at that moment. As weak as she became, she still had these incidents. Only rarely did she actually indicate that she was in pain, but her breathing became very shallow and labored. She ate nothing and would often not take her medications. Often these bouts of not eating and weakening were later found to be linked to an infection that had gone undiagnosed until it reached an acute stage. Somehow, with all of the recurrences of urinary tract infections and upper respiratory infections, no connection was ever made between the onset of behavioral symptoms and the start of an actual physical infection. Joan still wonders whether this connection, which persisted from the first months after the stroke to the last infection diagnosed a week before her death, could have been better monitored.

In keeping with her behavior when she lived in Florida, Ruth made no effort to develop relationships or even speak with other residents, many of whom were themselves not very communicative because of their own physical and cognitive frailty. When one of us asked her whether she knew any of the people around her she said something like, "I am a snob; I'd rather not socialize. Of course I would be cordial but I wouldn't want to be too close." She did, however, appreciate the aides and nurses who were kind to her. She especially liked the floor secretary, a young woman who often sat with her at lunch and patiently coaxed her to eat a little.

The staff treated Ruth with great kindness and very attentive care. In the last two weeks of her life, they were exceptional, speaking and handling our mother gently and answering all of Joan's questions patiently. Joan often remarked on how difficult it must be for the staff to watch all their patients eventually die, since few people enter a nursing home with an expectation of getting better and leaving. The staff was as kind to us as they were to our mother. They were at once highly professional and extremely compassionate. They seemed to sense that our mother was fading and they responded to the needs of her family. But above all, they tried to do anything they could to make Ruth more comfortable.

Her terminal event began with trouble breathing. It was never clear whether she had aspirated something or developed pneumonia or whether her congestive heart failure simply got worse. Perhaps she suffered a recurrence of her frequent urinary tract infections. Her x-ray looked like pneumonia. She stopped eating or taking food. The doctor called us and proposed putting her on an IV and giving her antibiotics. Although Ruth's advance directives clearly indicated that she did not want any heroic measures taken, and despite our recognition that the quality of her life had diminished to the point where there was little left, we chose to give her a chance to respond to this modest therapy. Although we had discussed many times the desirability of letting nature take its course, when the moment came, we could not simply concede without at least some modest effort. She did not respond to this treatment and we were decided against any further heroic measures, such as parenteral feeding or a nasogastric tube. Ruth was quite confused at the end, but when she woke for a moment quite agitated, the nurse tried to reassure her by saying, "You're all right, Ruth." Our mother looked at her with her last lucid glance and replied, "Like hell I am!" She died shortly thereafter, having "under-lived" her remaining assets by thirteen months. She died on May 29, four months and one week after she entered Sincerecare. When Joan and her husband returned to see her after her death, they both noted that she looked more peaceful than she had looked since her stroke three years earlier.

LESSONS

1   Even good nursing homes are institutions. They operate according to fixed rules and are very careful to stay within the accepted regulations.

2   Nursing home quality varies widely. Some information is posted on the Internet. The Medicare Web site called Nursing Home Compare offers some information about every nursing home in the country, but it certainly does not tell the whole story.

3   It is essential to shop carefully for the right nursing home. Gathering information is important but actually seeing the place is critical. Try the nose test: If it smells like feces and urine, get out. If it smells like disinfectant, beware; too much may be sacrificed to achieve cleanliness. But if it smells like chicken soup, this could be the place.

4   Few nursing homes are places to live; some are places only to die. Almost none provides a life-style that anyone would seek out.

5   Even good nursing homes continue to build double rooms despite the growing evidence that most older people want private rooms. The industry insists that double rooms are more cost effective, but those costs can be written off over long periods. Moreover, some studies suggest that the savings from reduced infection rates and

the need for less supervision with single-room occupancy more than offset these costs.

6   Informal caregiving, the jargon for family care (see Chapter 9), never stops, even after a person enters a nursing home

7   Residents whose family members visit regularly do better than those who have few visitors. The family may not always appreciate the importance of these visits because they are there to see the ultimate failures in care. Even the most curmudgeonly do not really want to be alone in their last days.

8   Nursing home staffs are more likely to pay closer attention to residents whose family is around and observing.

9   Nursing home residents need active family advocates. Like it or not, squeaky wheels do get the grease.

10   No matter how "out of it" a person with dementia seems, moments of lucidity are possible. People who look as though they are moribund can be roused by individual attention, though such responses are hard to predict.

11   Most group exercises for persons with dementia, watching videos and the like, which are the fare of activity programs, do not work well. Not everyone wants to be entertained. Not everyone finds being in a group pleasant.

Doctors, Other Medical Personnel, and Hospitals

Any frail older person will have plenty of encounters with the health care system. Indeed, medical care use is heavily skewed. A small number of individuals (perhaps 20 percent of the population) accounts for the majority (more than 70 percent) of all use. Not surprisingly, frail older persons are a large part of that 20 percent.

Frail older persons present special challenges to the health care system. In contrast to younger people, they rarely have a single problem. Indeed, a new problem is superimposed on all the old ones, often making it very difficult to detect just what is going on. Because aging is associated with decreased bodily responses to many stressors, in older people in general, and frail ones in particular, the usual signs and symptoms of disease, which might point clinicians in the right direction, are masked. For example, they may not run a fever with an infection or complain of pain with a heart attack. The symptoms they do have may be vague, such as agitation, confusion, or stupor. Like children, older people can quickly become dehydrated and develop confusion, even coma, as a result. Many clinicians are not familiar with the unusual ways disease can present in older patients, and medical schools teach little about geriatrics.

At the same time, older people are hard to treat because of communication problems. They may be hard of hearing or confused and unable to give a clear history. As the pressures to deliver care in ever shorter blocks of time conflict with the difficulties of obtaining a simple straightforward medical history and the complications of diagnosing disease in an older patient, many clinicians become frustrated. Few seem prepared to invest the time to obtain a complete assessment and to communicate their findings in a manner that the older patient can understand.

Frequently older patients are brought to busy emergency rooms (ERs) where their usual condition is not known and where the hectic pace and the general buzz of activity may agitate them even more. Few ER physicians have the time or temperament to work with confused older patients. ERs are stressful places for older people. One numerous occasions Ruth was left alone, lying in a gurney confused and frightened for long periods while more urgent cases were being treated.

Frail older persons and their families thus find themselves in a difficult position. They are very dependent on the medical care system but often find that system unresponsive and the personnel impatient. Sadly, those who need it most may find medical care hardest to use effectively. Even family members may be cowed by the dependency they feel on the system. Criticisms (including well-meant suggestions) that might alienate the few beacons of help and support they cling to are repressed

During the course of Ruth's illness, many people in hospital, clinical, office, and therapy settings exhibited real kindness and interest in her and in us. From May 1999 until her death three years later, she was seen by three different primary care physicians and three psychiatrists, as well as two dentists, various therapists, and dozens of nurses and aides from her various hospitalizations. Most of these people tried to respond constructively to her condition and to her needs. Yet, there were numerous times when the medical personnel sorely lacked the interpersonal skills to deal effectively and kindly with both Ruth and her family.

Our experience made it clear to us that hospitals do not operate for the well-being of the patient. They are institutions with rules and regulations that supercede the needs of the patients. Over a three-year period, Ruth was in at least seven hospital emergency rooms, resulting in stays for as little as twenty-four hours to as much as three weeks. Her condition at the time was always complicated by her bouts of agitation or the sun-downing syndrome common to most elderly demented patients. In every case, except one stay on a psychiatric ward, the treatment included giving her large doses of sedatives that would induce sleep and leave her totally dazed, confused, and even worse off than before the medication was administered. Much of the rationale for "doping her up" was that she could not be managed. Ruth would often not wait patiently to be toileted, and the hospital personnel wanted at all costs to prevent her falling "on their watch.". To keep her from becoming overly medicated we were compelled to hire our own private aides and thus to repeat the cycle referred to previously where she would become dependent on the attention, company, and assistance, making it hard to give up the extra aides once she returned to the assisted-living settings.

Because assisted-living facilities are risk averse and very conscious of being accused of neglect, Ruth made countless trips to ER facilities, usually precipitated by injuries (or simply fear of one) from a fall. Ruth also had serious problems with edema in her legs, which resulted in the formation of oozing sores that often required a trip to the ER for stitches and then a return for suture removal. Sometimes a visit to the ER was combined with a follow-up visit with her primary care physician or the nurse practitioner.

Although we went to great lengths to identify geriatricians who could oversee Ruth's care, we were unable to insure continuity of care. When most emergencies occurred either these physicians were not available or the ambulance summoned would insist on taking her to the nearest hospital, where the geriatrician did not have a clinical appointment.

By the fall of 2000 Ruth was being cared for by a doctor and a nurse practitioner who worked out of a university hospital-affiliated clinic. We felt confident that if Ruth should again be hospitalized the proximity of the two locations would work to our advantage. But it certainly did not on one day that still stands out as one of our most frustrating encounters with red tape and hospital "inhospitality."

The ER staff refused to page Ruth's doctor at the clinic. Joan had taken Ruth to the ER to get stitches removed, and at the same time Ruth's primary care physician wanted to see her to check on the latest bout of edema in her legs. Joan thought this would be an easy day, since she could take care of both issues in the same setting.

The ER staff, however, had a policy that they would not page doctors. Joan's insistence that the doctor had told her to have them page him made no difference. The only thing they would do was to give Joan an appointment in the clinic two hours later (but with a different physician, actually a medical student completely unfamiliar with both Ruth and her condition) so that Ruth could be seen for the edema. Joan had no choice but to keep Ruth in the hospital confined in a wheelchair without anyone to help her take Ruth to the bathroom. Ruth would often become like "dead weight" when Joan tried to transfer her, probably because she felt insecure and lacked faith that Joan could hold her easily. Her distrust and fear only aggravated Joan's lack of confidence in her ability to manage these transfers. This occurred at a time when Ruth was obsessed with using the bathroom very frequently. They waited over an hour beyond the scheduled appointment time and were finally seen by a well-intentioned but totally inexperienced young doctor, who finally went off in search of a mentoring doctor. At that precise moment, Ruth's regular doctor and the nurse practitioner happened to walk by and hear Joan's voice. They stuck their heads into the exam room and asked Joan why she and Ruth were there and not in the module where the doctor usually saw them and why Joan had not had them paged. By that point Joan was utterly frustrated and at a loss to understand why the ER personnel had been unwilling to even try paging them.

Several minutes later Joan was wheeling Ruth out of the clinic when she was stopped by a receptionist, who said that she was not yet free to go. He told Joan to get in line to see the cashier. There were at least eight people in the line. Joan explained that Ruth was in the system, that she, Joan, was on record as the one responsible for the bill, and that she was not checking out with the cashier. Ruth had long passed the point of being calm and patient. When he hesitated, Joan added that she would have a meltdown if he did not let her get Ruth out of there. He stepped back and let her go. With one simple electronic page, which the doctor had instructed Joan to ask for, the whole episode, lasting over five hours, might have taken twenty minutes.

Experiences like Joan's are all too common, and they are especially frustrating and upsetting when the patient is elderly, frail, disoriented, and confused. Over and over, the nonmedical personnel we encountered (receptionists and secretaries, acting as the "front line") seemed to lack any understanding of how difficult it can be to negotiate a medical facility, especially during a time of crisis and with a loved one who is suffering.

Sometimes nurses and doctors did try to accommodate Ruth. When she developed a small hernia, for example, the general surgeon agreed to do the repair with only local anesthesia when we explained how poorly she did in a hospital setting. He treated us all with dignity and kindness. The ophthalmologist who did the retina repair came at midnight to suture Ruth's eye and was patient in answering our questions and addressing our concerns. Unfortunately, the follow-up care was another instance of the staff's ordering Ativan or Haldol to calm our mother when she got restless.

During the three years Ruth spent in New York, post stroke, she had three primary care physicians. The first, who specialized in pulmonary care, seemed like an old-fashioned doctor. He was the most low key in the sense that he did not encourage invasive tests or procedures and though he had difficulty adjusting Ruth's medications, he would intercede if the hospital staff overmedicated her and he understood the need to get her off a urinary catheter before infections developed and muscle weakness set in.

When the pulmonary specialist died, his partner was not willing to take Ruth on. Robert arranged for a new doctor, a certified geriatrician who was interested and well intentioned and who tried to avoid hospitalizing Ruth. His office was extremely busy, however, and the waiting times were often difficult to negotiate with Ruth. She would become loud and angry in the waiting room and then revert to her pussycat charm when in the doctor's presence. The nurses were always the first to see her but she clearly preferred to be in the company of the male doctor. An office visit often took several hours, most of which was spent waiting. These delays increased the tension for Joan, who was always sensitive to how our mother's outbursts and comments were affecting the other patients and the office staff. The actual care and medical attention were not the issue. It was all of the attendant issues. The third physician was the head of geriatrics at the university hospital. She was very thorough and obliging when she saw Ruth but had many competing responsibilities. Much of Ruth's primary care was provided by the NP who worked closely with the geriatrician. This NP did make regular visits to Sunset.

Not all of the encounters with physicians were negative. Whenever sores appeared in Ruth's mouth from her dentures, for example, Joan's dentist always saw her promptly and the office staff were pleasant and helpful. Often, if the adjustment were slight, he would not even take money. And when Ruth was in the rehabilitation hospital and talking about wanting to die, a staff psychiatrist stayed with or near her over the Memorial Day weekend to provide continuous support and oversight to avoid using strong sedatives. She spent countless hours talking to our mother and to us and worked to find a combination of drugs that would improve Ruth's mood and attitude while allowing her to function in the rehabilitative environment.

At one point Joan took Ruth to her own primary care physician, whose office was more convenient. The doctor herself helped Ruth and Joan out to the car, where she and a member of her office staff helped transfer Ruth into the car. That act of kindness remains etched in Joan's memory, reminding her that she did indeed encounter some very compassionate, caring medical people along the journey of our mother's post-stroke life. Joan still recalls her overwhelming sense of gratitude for the slightest unexpected act of random kindness that was bestowed on our mother.

It is a sad commentary that such an experience is so memorable because it was rare. Kindness and consideration should be routine. Family members greatly appreciate help with tasks like getting wheelchairs in and out of cars, but few office staff members seem to even recognize the problem, let alone offer assistance.

By contrast, some nurses and receptionists showed their annoyance when Joan asked for their assistance transferring Ruth in or out of the car. Because Ruth did not have confidence in Joan's ability to hold her securely, she would stiffen up or become very angry or agitated and uncooperative, causing Joan to feel even more uncomfortable about asking for help.

Joan's own dentist was also particularly kind to our mother. Whenever sores appeared in Ruth's mouth from her dentures, he always saw her promptly and the office staff were pleasant and lovely about helping. Often, if the adjustment were slight, he would not even take money.

In almost every hospital setting, we had difficulty dealing with the business staff. Although they were often very well intentioned, they were usually hampered by understaffing, and many lacked the personal skills of empathy and compassion necessary to respond appropriately to patients who are old, disoriented, and seemingly demanding. Some were inflexible and very hard to deal with. Also, the extensive bureaucratic paperwork (on the computer) required for reimbursement and the lines of patients waiting to register were difficult for us to negotiate, as they would be for anyone accompanying a frail, sick, or elderly person. Often office workers sorely lacked the personal skills of empathy and compassion. They were sometimes inflexible and very difficult to deal with.

Ruth had no concept of time and was unable to postpone gratification. However unrealistic, she demanded attention immediately. It often seemed that even one more aide per unit would have made a huge difference in the care and attention that was provided. With better administration, the actual contact time with the patients in all aspects of hospital care would increase. Perhaps the need for so many sedating drugs might be reduced, if not eliminated.

This variation in basic hospital care was especially evident during the hospitalization after the fall that disturbed the stitches in Ruth's cornea. On Sunday, a day when many usual hospital activities did not occur, the staff was very attentive. But by Monday, the staff was once again caught up in the busy rhythm of diagnosis and treatment and ignored our mother, who was by now no longer in acute danger. Not only was there no pleasant chatting but the staff clearly viewed her as an inconvenience and a very low priority.

On many occasions, after we had seen that our mother was settled in the room and after having emphasized with the nursing staff the difficult reactions our mother had to psychoactive medications, we left with assurances that no sedatives would be used. Nonetheless, we would return in the morning to find Ruth unable to wake up from drugs administered during the night. Not only was it upsetting for us, but more important, it was usually the start of a decline for our mother. She would leave the hospital in worse shape than when she entered.

Older patients, especially those with dementia, can readily become objects instead of people. One of the horrible memories of the night Ruth was rushed to the ER for repair of the stitches in her cornea is of the discussion we had in the preoperative hall with the anesthesiologist and the ophthalmologist's assistants about the fact that DNR (do not resuscitate) orders are suspended during surgery. We were talking in the third person about Ruth's life while she lay on a stretcher insisting she wanted to urinate. There is something terribly sad and troubling about the way our mother was depersonalized. Undoubt-edly the stresses associated with bouts of illness and all of the logisti-cal problems that these crises precipitated made our reactions more acute, but most hospital care occurs in response to just such events. A compassionate medical care system must be able to deal with these exigencies.

In many instances the professionals involved were more support-ive and compassionate than those who dealt with the public. The medical care system has erected a series of checkpoints. The gate-keepers who control access to care often seemed highly insensitive to patients' conditions and issues. Perhaps they saw it as part of their job to protect the busy schedules of the professionals, perhaps the pressure of maintaining the pace of care flow was simply too much, but their manner exacerbated the whole situation. More at-tention to this critical interface with the public could go a long way to improving care and reducing the inevitable stress that caring for a frail person induces in both the professional caregivers and the patient's family.

Although most of the doctors and health care professionals were polite and reasonably responsive to Joan, they made it apparent from the beginning that they preferred to speak directly to Robert, the physician son, in almost all instances, even if the information was not highly technical. Once any physician found out one of the patient's children was a doctor, the pattern was quickly established for Robert to intervene and call the doctor directly. Our case may have been further complicated by Robert's prominence as a geriatric researcher, which meant the doctors wanted to be especially careful to run everything by him first. Some of the doctors were almost dismissive of Joan and insisted on speaking with Robert long distance. This direct communication did work to Joan's advantage, however, to the extent that it meant she did not have to go through all of the gatekeepers and preliminary waiting on hold to speak to the doctor.

The only exception to this prejudice toward Joan was the ophthalmologist, who usually did not ask to confer with Robert. He was very clear and direct in articulating the medical situations to Joan, although she sometimes requested that certain questions be funneled through Robert. Although we always discussed issues and choices openly with one another and agreed on all decisions, there were clearly times when the Joan could see she was not part of the medical "club." Communicating with doctors is generally hard for lay persons. The doctors do not return telephone calls from lay people promptly and sometimes lay people are put on hold for long periods when they call a doctor's office. Doctors calling other doctors, however, are generally treated with much more deference. Calls are returned quickly. Waiting times on hold are shorter. Part of this difference may be the result of professional courtesy, but when it implies a lack of concern for the families of all patients it is troubling.

LESSONS

1   Hospitals seem to function more for the convenience of the doctors and the staff than the patients and their families.
2   It is inhumane for frail, confused, old people to be taken to the hospital and left alone on stretchers. It is a frightening, disorienting experience for anyone, but so much the worse for this population.

3   Hospitals are understaffed and prone to error. Most errors happen not because of incompetence but because of carelessness.

4   Hypervigilance is crucial. You cannot assume that hospitals will not make careless mistakes. You cannot afford to be cowed. You must be willing to ask questions and to challenge what seem to be errors.

5   Because hospitals are often short staffed, it is easy to ignore patients, particularly those who are frail and older, who do not have critical problems. Hence, such people should be discharged as quickly as possible, and when they are there, they need advocates to insist that they get the attention they need and deserve.

6   Medical care seems very inefficient. Often the same questions are asked over and over, as if no one is aware of or trusts the information others have just obtained. Better information systems are needed that allow accurate data to be shared more effectively.

7   Nurse practitioners who can work closely with physicians can make medical care much more effective and responsive.

8   Office and other hospital workers should be better trained to deal more humanely with patients and their caregivers.

9   The scheduling of doctors' appointments must be improved so that elderly, frail people do not have to sit and wait for long periods. They do not tolerate the waits well and may disrupt waiting rooms.

10   Many doctors do not communicate information readily and may talk down to patients and their family; they respond very differently to other doctors.

11   Doctors are not always rational, and medical practice may be driven by fear of litigation. Most physicians now recognize that many families have access to lots of information on the Internet and elsewhere. In some places the nature of the doctor-patient relationship is changing as a result. Doctors may become annoyed when confronted by families who have looked up information on the Internet.

12   Doctors know much less than we think they do; some are optimists and some are pessimists. It is important to ask them for the evidence on which they are basing their prognoses. Unfortunately not all doctors welcome being challenged. A physician who is uncomfortable explaining why he or she is doing something may not really know why. Be tactful, even deferential, but be persistent.

13   Medicine is still not based primarily on hard evidence. Much of it is based on judgments. Furthermore, practice patterns and the definition of appropriate medical care vary widely. What is considered good care in one place may not be in another. Do not hesitate to ask for a second opinion.

14   Clinical variation is a hallmark of aging. Problems do not present the same way in older persons as they do in younger ones. Not all physicians, indeed not many physicians, are well trained in geriatrics. Few older patients are classic cases that fit neatly into conventional wisdom. Physicians may miss subtle or atypical signs and symptoms.

Informal Care

nformal care, which is jargon in the gerontological literature for the unpaid care of family and friends, is the heart of long-term care. Most informal care is supplied by women—wives, daughters, and daughters-in-law. Many observers have worried that as more and more women enter the workforce, the availability of this critical informal care will diminish sharply. So far there has been no sign of such a diminution. As our story illustrates, women simply (perhaps not so simply) add to their already busy schedules a new set of tasks.

One might expect that using institutional care would obviate the need for much of the informal care that is central to allowing a frail older person to remain at home. Although many of the daily personal care burdens are relieved by institutionalization, the intensity of informal care support remains high, and the emotional burdens are at least as great. Once a frail older person is institutionalized, the family member who has been totally in control of personally delivered care becomes dependent on the actions of others to provide this care. For some, such delegation can be difficult.

One of the reasons respite care has not been as widely embraced as many had expected may well be that those who provide intensive informal care have great difficulty relinquishing their role. Perhaps the only way they can sustain the enormous burden that such care imposes, especially in the care of demented persons, is to consider themselves irreplaceable. Accepting respite would mean admitting that someone else can step into that role, if only temporarily.

This chapter is recounted largely through the eyes of our mother's principal caregiver, her daughter, Joan. During most of the period of this narrative Joan was employed full-time as an elementary school teacher with heavy commitments to meet her class schedule. Also during this period her first two grandchildren were born on the opposite coast, and she wanted to spend as much time as possible with them.

Joan's role as the informal caregiver changed with each transition in our mother's care. The task was difficult from the onset in the hospital just after her stroke. In an intensive care unit (ICU) there is very little family members are allowed to actually do for a post-stroke patient, but Ruth was highly sensitive to certain stimuli, in particular to the feeling of the sheet on her body if it was not perfectly smooth. Thus began the first test of how well we would be able to meet our mother's needs. She was verbally abusive and alternated between demanding our presence at her bedside and calling us names and insisting we had not made her covers straight enough. Sadly, no amount of pulling and tugging could satisfy and calm her.

Most of our caregiving at that stage was confined to providing emotional support and acting as her advocate with the hospital personnel. In effect, we became her agents, making critical decisions in her stead. We stayed by her bedside trying to make her comfortable but could provide little in the way of actual service.

The need for continuous informal care was one of the major reasons we transferred our mother from Florida to New York when she was ready for discharge from the ICU. We realized that she had little or no informal support in Florida. Joan, who had always been solicitous to her needs, was prepared to play an active role in her care.

From the moment Ruth entered rehabilitation, Joan had great difficulty setting the boundaries for how much care she needed to provide for her. Part of the difficulty was due to Joan's personality. She freely acknowledges that she feels a sense of responsibility to take care of people and situations. Joan has been known to feel the need to help strangers who cry out for help in hospitals; so it is no great surprise that she felt driven to do anything she could to help her own mother.

Joan's work hours meant that she could not visit our mother until almost four or five in the afternoon. Hospitals are happy to have family around to assist patients with eating, but in rehab the rules are stricter. Ruth was expected to eat in the communal dining room, but if Joan was there at dinnertime, Ruth would often refuse to go to the dining room with the other patients. She was very reluctant to participate in any of the social group functions, including meals in the dining room. Joan would often wheel her in, try to get her settled, and then leave so she would be forced to adapt. For Ruth, any visit from her daughter was an excuse for her not to join others in routine activities, and her participation became erratic and unpredictable.

At Terraceview, the first assisted-living facility Ruth moved to, it was the family's job to do laundry, organize the room, and provide the amenities necessary to make her feel comfortable and at home. All of these responsibilities fell on Joan, who took them on willingly. In fact, whenever her visit was briefer than usual, she felt better knowing that at least she was doing all of these other things to take care of our mother. Ruth was very dependent on Joan for comfort and familiarity. She had not lived in the area for over twenty years; and no one else, other than Robert and his wife and occasionally a grandchild and ,Joan's husband, who was always there for the emergencies, ever visited her. But Joan was there every day for the first few months and almost every day until she could wean both her mother and herself to three times a week.

Joan would wash her mother's hair and blow it dry. Appearances were important to Ruth and she enjoyed the attention she always received for looking attractive and well groomed. Indeed, appearances are also important to Joan, perhaps because she was reared by a glamorous mother. The decline in Ruth's physical appearance was especially upsetting to Joan. Our mother had always taken great pride in her appearance. This once elegant woman, who had instilled similar values in Joan, was now perpetually messy, spilling, drooling, and soiling her clothing. Joan tried to keep her as neat as possible, frequently changing her clothes and ultimately buying very simple clothing that was easy to wash. Nonetheless, every meal was an invitation to disaster. Ruth was harder to keep clean than a two-year-old. The one saving grace was that her mind deteriorated too, so she was often unaware of how messy and dirty she was.

Joan's caregiving involved doing Ruth's laundry and shopping for drugs, cosmetics, clothes, snacks, and any other items she needed. To accommodate Ruth's feet, which swelled with episodic edema, Joan even found a shoe-store owner who made "house calls" to the assisted-living facility. Therapists came during the day to the assisted-living facility, but for all other appointments, Joan made dates in the late afternoon. For as long as Ruth was ambulatory, Joan would take her for manicures and pedicures after school. On many of these out-ings, the two of them would have dinner out or Joan would stay with Ruth while she ate a late meal in her room.

Even though Joan did not make it to the assisted-living facility every day, she had frequent telephone conversations with the staff and with Ruth, until her telephone was removed. Often in the evening Ruth became disoriented or sad, and she would call Joan, demanding hysterically that she come right over. Usually by the time Joan arrived, Ruth was calm again and had forgotten the call. Occasionally she would cry and insist that Joan sit there until she fell asleep.

At Terraceview we were paying for the highest level of care, which included help with showering, dressing and undressing, behavioral management, and toilet care. But the Terraceview staff often had called Joan to come over to calm Ruth down during a particularly bad bout of agitation or abusive behavior. Usually Joan could talk Ruth through the worst of these outbursts over the telephone, but not always. Sometimes she had to drive over in the middle of the night and try to settle her down.

In response to all these problems we decided that we needed to find part-time aides to keep our mother company. As described ear-lier, this part-time solution evolved into hiring a full-time aide. Once the full-time day aide was hired, Joan happily relinquished the laun-dry to her charge and never took back that job; the aide was able to use the washing machines on the premises. The aide also took charge of grooming Ruth, and so the need for Joan to shampoo and style her hair was gone as well. Joan still visited daily, but she felt a certain sense of relief that some of our mother's needs were being met by someone besides her. The aide could take Ruth to a doctor's appointment if such a visit could not be scheduled after school hours, and once she was even able to take her to the dentist for an emergency visit .

Each successive placement changed the amount of actual care Joan provided. After the move to Sunset, we no longer needed to hire an aide during the day. The facility's staff did the laundry and took care of all matters of personal hygiene were also handled by the aide. Ruth's routine health issues were handled by a nurse practitioner who made on- site visits. But as our mother's health declined and the number of falls increased, so did the frequency of trips to the emergency room (ER). Although Joan responded to most calls herself, sometimes her husband would leave work to handle things. At other times Sunset used ambulance services and Joan had to leave school to meet Ruth in the ER.

One episode during Ruth's stay at Sunset indicates the extent to which these institutions can be rigid and uncooperative. Ruth developed an eye infection on a Saturday when Joan was away for the weekend. Ruth's primary care physician insisted that she be seen by the eye specialist on Monday. In the meantime, she was to have her eyes washed out periodically with baby shampoo, a product that is available over the counter. Sunset was across the street from a large-chain pharmacy, but no one could be dispatched to buy the shampoo, even though Joan offered to pay for the shampoo and the time involved, explaining by telephone that for her to buy and deliver it would necessitate a long drive. An aide could have stopped there on a break; an administrator could have run over; any worker could have done the favor after hours. Instead, Joan had to call upon a friend to travel eight miles out of her way to deliver the baby shampoo. It was hard to understand the rationale for refusing to accommodate Joan, who consistently made every effort to meet all of Sunset's requests promptly.

No matter what services were provided by the institutions where Ruth spent the last three years of her life, nothing took the place of visits from family, particularly her children. When Ruth first came to New York, Robert flew in every couple of months or if the condition worsened, as well as the few times when Joan left for a vacation or to visit her grandchildren across the country. As Ruth's condition worsened, he came more often. Grandchildren would visit whenever they arrived in New York, but these visits were rare. Of Ruth's five grandchildren, only three actually saw her during her illness. She also had six great-grandchildren, two of whom were born during that period. Several of her great-grandchildren were able to visit her. She seemed to be interested in hearing about the births but did not respond to photographs of great-grandchildren or to other photographs of her extended family. The staff at Sunset encouraged the use of photographs to help orient residents to their rooms. Looking back, we realize that perhaps we should have given Ruth childhood pictures of her and her parents and sister. It is hard to accept that the great-grandchildren were a blur. One, whom she never met, was named for her in the month before her death. When Ruth's grandchildren brought their children to visit, she responded to the babies, but really just as babies with no sense that they were related to her. She did, however, seem to recognize her grandchildren and was pleased to see them.

Joan would try to see our mother a minimum of three times a week, but there was a constant pall hanging over her. The visits usually lasted no more than an hour. Rarely could Ruth sustain a real conversation and the same few questions were asked and answered over and over. On mild days, Joan would take her outside on the terrace, where most times, she would doze off. Some days Ruth would be grateful for the sight of Joan's face but then become concerned about how much time she was spending and tell her to go. Other days, if she was agitated, even Joan's arrival would not soothe her and drugs were used to calm her down. Joan would leave feeling elated after a pleasant visit and profoundly sad after a difficult encounter. But because Ruth's moods were so unpredictable, Joan was constantly on edge and it was often easier to suffer the guilt of not going rather than risk disappointment and terrible sadness if a visit went badly.

Even prior to Ruth's stroke, when it became clear that her mental status was deteriorating, Joan had become a co-signator on her bank account and had assumed power of attorney for other financial arrangements. She continued to manage her affairs after her illness, paying all the bills using our mother's funds. Until her death, our mother's resources were sufficient to pay for her own care.

The caregiving experience during Ruth's illness was different for each of us, in part because of the different roles we took on and in part because of the historical relationship we each had with our mother. Joan bore most of the burden, being on call every day. Indeed, she had always been more attentive to our mother. Long before Ruth's health began to deteriorate, Joan would call daily and make sure that her needs were met. She would bring Ruth to New York to visit regularly. When Joan's two boys were growing up, Ruth had played an active role as a grandmother and had formed close attachments to them. Her relationship to Robert was quite different. He was her golden-haired boy, a doctor and a professor. She delighted in bragging about, and exaggerating, his accomplishments. Robert called her much less frequently and visited several times a year, usually in combination with a business trip. She rarely saw his children, except on special family occasions, although they would make special efforts to visit her as they grew older. Whereas Ruth was quick to criticize Joan's appearance, whenever she saw Robert, she exclaimed over how handsome he looked. When Ruth became ill, Robert played a dual role. As a geriatrician, he became the overseer of her medical care and other aspects of her formal care. He used his contacts and reputation to leverage the best care available. As her son, he spent two intensive weeks at her side immediately after the stroke and through her transfer to the rehabilitation hospital in New York. Thereafter his visits were much less frequent, precipitated by a crisis or a need to provide some coverage or coincident with a business trip to the vicinity. He was in daily communication with Joan, providing both advice and support. All decisions were made jointly.

Partly because of his professional training and partly because his visits were infrequent, Robert tried to encourage Ruth to be as active as possible. He would walk with her and take her out for meals and short trips. When he was in town he would spend long days with her, keeping her stimulated. Initially these sojourns were very effective, but as her condition declined it became increasingly difficult to mobilize her. It took the fiasco of her last trip outside, the attempt to get pizza, to convince Robert that it was no longer feasible to take Ruth out for a meal.

As Ruth's cognitive state deteriorated Robert called her less frequently, feeling that it was a waste because the conversation would immediately be forgotten and anyway, he had never been comfortable chatting on the telephone. Often, however, he got credit for calls he had never made because Ruth simply imagined them, and imagined contact seemed to be as much appreciated as real contact. Indeed, the value of regular contact, especially by telephone, is a subject of debate in the literature on dementia care. While Ruth was in the nursing home, Robert did get his first cell phone to keep himself in easy contact with Joan and Ruth's doctors about her condition while he was away.

Giving care in short bursts as Robert did is a totally different experience from being there day in and day out as Joan was. It is the difference between a sprinter and a marathoner. But we both felt the stress of caregiving and it brought us closer together. We talked on the telephone several times a week, much more than we ever had done before Ruth's stroke. An important reason for contact was to provide psychological support for Joan, who bore the daily brunt of care and was more emotionally invested in what was happening; but we also needed to discuss concerns and plans. We became committed to a common cause and struggled with what we could do to minimize the tragedy we saw unfolding before us.

The closer we became to each other, the more stress developed with our respective spouses, who, in such a situation, were bound to be excluded. Although Robert's wife was a gerontologist and long-term-care expert in her own right, her efforts to be helpful were not always well received. As Robert was struggling to juxtapose the theory he had taught with the reality he was experiencing, he often found his wife's suggestions unrealistic. To Joan those suggestions sounded like criticisms of what she was trying to do or what she believed. Indeed, what were likely many valid observations and useful suggestions went unheeded because we both interpreted them as criticisms.

We disagreed about some financial issues. Although we had agreed to jointly support Ruth after her own resources ran out, Joan was prepared before that point to spend whatever was needed to provide Ruth with every comfort. If twenty-four-hour nursing care was suggested, she was ready to agree to it. Robert, by contrast, wanted to push harder for more services from the various institutions that were already being paid to provide service. He was concerned that huge expenses up front would deplete Ruth's resources unnecessarily. We discussed her finances quite openly. Neither of us was especially concerned about preserving (or creating) a legacy from Ruth's finances, and, although we realized that the money spent on her care would not be available to support our own grandchildren, for whom we had both taken steps to provide educational funds.

As long as assisted living met Ruth's needs, neither of us raised the issue of seeking advice on how to reassign her assets to make her eligible for Medicaid. Medicaid held no allure because it does not cover this form of care. Only when it became clear that Ruth would have to go to a nursing home did we begin to explore Medicaid.

LESSONS

1   The need for informal family caregiving does not stop when a frail elderly person moves to a congregate care setting, even a nursing home.

2   Although the need for informal care never stops, it is essential that the primary caregiver take a break. No one wins when the primary caregiver burns out.

3   The burden of informal care usually falls on one person, though other family members are often actively involved.

4   Family members should clarify and agree on the overall goals of the care being sought. Even those who take a smaller role in the care process may have strong opinions that will be disruptive if they are not voiced and discussed.

5   To avoid feelings of resentment, family members should be aware that not all siblings make good caregivers and that therefore equity is not always the best basis for assigning roles. Do not ask those who cannot give to do their share. It is a losing proposition. Sometimes you can identify tasks (even contributing financially) that family memberswho do not have the temperament for direct care can perform.

6   Informal caregiving comes in many forms: providing personal services (e.g., bathing, grooming, dressing), transportation, emotional support, and financial support, doing chores (e.g., laundry, shopping), managing finances, serving as an advocate, and just being there. Ideally, each person should contribute according to what he or she can do best. Inevitably some family members will do more than others, and it is important to acknowledge this discrepancy. Nonetheless, it is usually important to clarify the overall goals of the care being sought. Even those who do not contribute much to the care process may have strong opinions that will disrupt things if they are not voiced and discussed.

7   Patterns of informal care are often shaped by previous relationships with the care recipient. In the stress of providing care, unresolved issues inevitably emerge.

8   Patterns of caregiving differ according to whether the service is performed regularly or infrequently.

9   Informal caregiving takes a heavy toll on the primary caregiver. Research studies show that informal caregivers suffer disproportionately from stress-related illness. But often caregivers become so focused and intent on doing the job that they do not recognize the effect the whole experience is having until after it is all over. Caregivers therefore should be sensitive to signs of stress in themselves and be prepared to get help with the caregiving and with the stress.

10   Caregiving cannot be wholly unselfish. A good caregiver must protect himself or herself, if only to continue giving the care. It is foolish to enter into a situation where you know it will demand more than is feasible. It is hard enough to do what you believe to be the right thing. Martyrs have short half-lives.

11   Avoid early burnout. Caregiving needs marathoners not sprinters. You need to pace yourself for the long haul.

The Roads Not Taken

During our mother's illness, we made decisions that had particularly great consequences for the future. Each such decision meant choosing one option and forgoing another. There is no test to determine whether a decision is good or not, only the constant reassessment of an outcome experienced. Life is not a series of opportunities to go down each path, and in the end, we had to be satisfied with having done our best to consider as many of the consequences as we could imagine for each choice.

Ruth's stated preference, after her stroke, was to stay at home in Florida, and once we made the decision to move her to New York, she wanted to have her own new home there. Later, she did not like the dementia unit in the assisted-living facility and regularly pleaded with Joan to take her home or set her up in an apartment. Like Ruth, most older people strongly prefer to stay in their own home, especially when the alternative is something akin to a nursing home. However, many older persons are now voluntarily moving into assisted-living facilities, which allow them to give up the responsibilities of maintaining a household while retaining control over most aspects of their own lives. It is not surprising that more women than men are making this choice. Women usually outlive their partners and they are the ones who must do most of the household chores that, with increasing age and frailty, can become burdensome.

We never entertained for long the idea that our mother could manage on her own, or even with help, in Florida. Admittedly we made decisions quite early in the course of her stroke, before we knew just how well she would fare after rehabilitation. But the risk was simply too great. Leaving her to recuperate in Florida would have meant that one of us would have had to suspend normal life for a sustained period, oversee her rehabilitative care, arrange for follow-up care, and oversee that care for several weeks or even months. Both of us had active commitments to our respective work. Negotiating a sustained leave of absence would have been extremely difficult.

Having made the decision to transfer our mother to New York, we discussed the feasibility of setting her up in an apartment with twenty-four-hour help once she completed rehabilitation. The costs would likely have been equivalent to those entailed in assisted living, especially once we started paying for private-duty aides. We did not pursue this option for several reasons:

- The residual responsibility involved in insuring continuity of care would fall on Joan, who was already working full time.
- The stability of the arrangement would require a great deal of oversight and maintenance. Even if we could recruit someone to live in and provide twenty-four-hour care, we would at least need to arrange some coverage for days off.

- The likelihood of achieving a stable relationship between Ruth and a caregiver was very low. Our mother tolerated strangers very badly and her fits of pique would quickly alienate even the kindest workers. Dealing with her when she became anxious and subject to outbursts could be very taxing

The situation might have been different if Ruth already had established a household in Long Island. Returning someone to a familiar environment is easier than setting up a new one. Because she would not be returning to an already established residence, it would mean setting up a living situation from scratch.

Keeping a family member at home who is in need of care raises a variety of concerns in addition to the basic logistics. It means trusting a stranger to have total and virtually unsupervised control over your family member. In an assisted-living facility, even if supervision is lax, there is some sense of accountability and oversight that is absent in a home care arrangement. Contracting with an agency might offer some of this oversight, but it would make the proposition very expensive, and even then the supervision would be cursory at best, although the agency might provide some reassurance of backup services and prior screening.

In addition to safety (and freedom from abuse) there are also fears about theft. In our mother's case, where we would be creating virtually a new household, there would likely be little to steal.

Before deciding to move Ruth to New York, we discussed the alternative of having her move to Minneapolis, where Robert lived. Care in Minnesota would have been much cheaper. Based on discussions with friends and colleagues in the long-term care business, we estimate that we could have bought at least as good if not better care for half to two-thirds the cost in New York. Moreover, the style of assisted living provided in Minnesota, at least in the private market, might have allowed Ruth to stay in that type of care longer.

There were several strong arguments against moving her to Minneapolis. Joan was the truly devoted caregiver and she would have had great difficulty not being able to attend to her mother. Robert would never have been as attentive, if only because his travel schedule would have meant his being away a great deal. Even more important, he did not have the temperament to spend long periods attending to her basic care needs. In the end the decision respected Joan's psychological need to be the primary caregiver and her aptitude for the role.

The geographic differences in care and coverage are important to recognize. Long-term care is largely a state issue. While private assisted living has flourished in many states, most have only modest coverage for this type of care under Medicaid. Where such coverage exists the care it provides is generally much less elegant than that purchased privately.

For Ruth, a potential missed opportunity was the purchase of long-term care insurance. When she was well into her eighties, she was besieged by insurance agents who wanted to sell her long-term care policies. These policies would have paid various amounts to offset the costs of long-term care. Some paid cash; some paid directly for services. Some were triggered by a given state of persistent disability, such as inability to care for herself for three months. Others used the actual use of services as the trigger. They might pay half or two-thirds of the cost after she paid the first part. In this way, they could limit their liability to cases where the person really was prepared to use formal services.

Robert urged Ruth not to buy any of these policies under the calculation that most would cover only modest amounts of service and that the likelihood of ever using enough benefits to offset the premium costs was low. Moreover, the primary rationale for long-term care insurance is to preserve assets, essentially to pass them on as a legacy. Neither Robert nor Joan had any strong need or desire for Ruth's assets. Both were content to see that the funds were used to support her.

In retrospect, long-term care insurance might have proven to be a wise investment. Depending on the policy, insurance might have covered at least part of her assisted-living costs. It would certainly have covered some of the costs of the aides we hired and a modest part of the costs of the nursing home.

As things worked out, Ruth's assets were sufficient to see her though her whole course of long-term care and still leave a modest inheritance. Her three years in long-term career cost about $330,000. The seventeen-month stay in Terraceview cost about $90,000 for the room and board and an additional $44,000 for the aides. Her fourteen-month stay at Sunset cost about $100,500 and an additional $34,000 for the aides. The four months in the nursing home cost $61,625.

When Ruth had the stroke she had about $430,000 in assets (including her condominium). When she died she had $100,000 left. Long-term care insurance would likely have increased that amount to about $210,000. Indeed, most long-term care insurance policies would have been about a break-even proposition, depending on their specific benefits and premiums. If she had bought a policy at age eighty, it would have cost about $2,000 a month or $24,000 a year. If she paid premiums for the four years until she needed long-term care, they would have cost $96,000. The policy would have paid out about $90,500 ($28,700 for the aides, at $50 a day; $46,500 for assisted living, at $50 a day; and $15,300 for nursing home, at $120 a day).

People in a situation similar to ours but with fewer assets would probably have been eligible for Medicaid. In most states, however, Medicaid does not usually cover assisted living, or at least not at the level of luxury Ruth was buying, and Medicaid does not allow the range of choice in assisted-living facilities we demanded. Nor does it pay additionally for private aides.

State Medicaid programs vary widely in their approach to covering assisted living. Some see it as a good buy, costing less than what they would pay for comparable nursing home care. Others see it as an added expense that can induce demand for such care. Where Medicaid does cover assisted living, it covers only the services portion. Room and board are supposed to be paid by Social Security income and special welfare supplements when needed. Most Medicaid spending goes to nursing homes, although many states will cover some forms of home care for persons who are judged to otherwise qualify for nursing home care.

For Ruth to become Medicaid eligible would have required our spending down her assets earlier than Ruth would have wanted. We chose not to explore asset divestiture until very late in her course. Estate planners counsel families about how to conserve or shelter an older person's assets in order to speed up their eligibility for Medicaid. Medicaid eligibility levels vary from state to state, but they are generally based on a combination of income and assets. While many older persons have modest incomes, they may have substantial assets that far exceed the very meager levels allowed by Medicaid.

Because we were determined to keep our mother out of a nursing home as long as possible and because Medicaid coverage of assisted living is generally poor, we saw no strong reason to engage in such asset sheltering, leaving aside considerations of the ethics of the practice. Ultimately, however, once it became clear that Ruth would need nursing home care, we did consult an attorney who specializes in this area and were advised to spend or transfer her assets down to a level that would legally entitle her to Medicaid assistance sometime in the future. As things turned out, she never lived long enough for us to confront that decision.

The ethics, legality, and extent of asset divestiture are hotly debated. While some observers see it as commonplace, efforts to quantify the phenomenon suggest it is much rarer than many believe. In part, this whole concept reflects a major change in public policy. For many years Medicaid was seen as a welfare program designed to cover the poor. But as long-term care has become a major expense for more and more American families, many middle-class people have come to view Medicaid as a right for them. They have paid taxes to support this program for years and feel that now it should help them. At least in this instance, the stigma of welfare has to some extent been expunged. It is no longer unusual to hear even upper-middle-class people talking about asset divestiture and Medicaid coverage.

Perhaps as more families experience the reality of long-term care, public sentiment will shift. People will come to see this aspect of care as worthy of greater attention. They will urge active debate on public policies that address all people at risk, not just the poor or the faux poor. If long-term care insurance makes sense, it makes the most sense as some sort of universal coverage that would make it both affordable and accessible to all. The difference between using Medicaid and having universal long-term care insurance is simply a matter of degree and commitment to sharing the burden and benefits equitably.

Ultimately we wound up making a whole series of decisions, some of which were predicated on ones we had made earlier. In addition to making medical decisions in emergencies, we had to decide:

- Whether Ruth would stay in Florida or move to be near one of us, and when she should leave Florida—before or after rehabilitation
- Which of us would be the primary caregiver and in what state—two interlinked decisions
- What kind of care Ruth needed—home care, assisted living, nursing home
- How much money we should spend
- Whether to transfer her assets to make her eligible for Medicaid
- How much private-duty help to buy and when
- When to establish and what to include in advance directives
- Whether to buy long-term care insurance (prior to her stroke)
- When to go on outings and when to stop taking Ruth out
- What end-of-life care Ruth should get

Looking back on all those decisions, there are few things we would have done differently. Perhaps it was foolish not to think about preserving more of her assets, but we were determined to keep her in assisted living as long as possible. Perhaps it would have been feasible to set her up in an apartment with round-the-clock help. The costs would likely not have been much more than what we ended up paying, but it would have placed an even heavier burden on Joan. Perhaps we should have moved her out of the first assisted-living facility sooner, but the inevitable disruption of transfer made it easy to delay that move.

The big unanswered question is whether our mother's life in the last three years was worthwhile to her. There certainly were moments when it seemed to us that it was, and others when it seemed it was not, especially for someone who so dreaded being dependent. Before her stroke Ruth had repeatedly said that she would rather be dead than disabled. But after the stroke she seemed to adapt to her disabled state and rarely spoke about wanting to die.

LESSONS

1   Many long-term care situations seem intolerable in the abstract, but some older persons seem to accept these situations once confronted with them. Many people say they would rather be dead than live severely disabled but they cling to life once they are disabled.

2   It is easy to leave the frail older person, who are the center of attention, out of the decision-making process, but that does not make it the right thing to do. It is critical to think about what the patient would want, but it is hard to know. At the same time, you cannot accede to all the requests from these patients, who almost always will insist that they can stay in their homes, even when such a choice is infeasible.

3   Life does not allow do-overs. It is important to make the best choices you can and then, for peace of mind, not to constantly reassess the consequences of every decision.

4   It is important to recognize which choices are likely to impose intolerable burdens. Doing the noble thing may not be good for anyone.

The End of Life

We discussed end-of-life care on many occasions, regularly lamenting that the end of our mother's life was not playing out as she had scripted it. Knowing how she dreaded being disabled, it was not difficult for us to interpret her desires concerning what she wanted done if she became even more incapacitated. In the two assisted-living facilities, Ruth eagerly completed advance directives that declared that no efforts should be made to resuscitate her. She filled out legalistic forms making Robert the person responsible for acting in her stead if she could no longer communicate.

Neither of us felt therefore that any heroic efforts should be made to sustain what had become a life with little quality. Indeed, we often spoke out loud of the blessing it would be if she died peacefully in her sleep. We even went on to plan her funeral, including discussing whether we would have one at all. Long before her stroke, Ruth had purchased and paid for a cremation program. Typically idiosyncratic and a bit dramatic, she wanted her ashes to be scattered at sea, rather than to be buried beside those of her husband, and she contracted with an organization called the Neptune Society for that purpose. She indicated that she did not want a formal funeral. We agreed with those wishes in principle but anticipated some sort of informal reception on her death and a more organized memorial service some time later when all the family could gather.

Given our agreement about what steps should be taken when the time came, one might expect that we were well prepared her eventual death. The reality, however, was different.

At the outset of what proved to be her terminal episode, Joan observed that Ruth was doing poorly. The nursing home staff initiated a basic evaluation and called Robert to discuss the situation. The geriatrician and Robert agreed that Ruth likely had an infection and was dehydrated. Although her advance directives clearly indicated that no active steps should be taken and her quality of life had diminished greatly over the past several months, it seemed reasonable nonetheless to give her the chance to benefit from at least modest treatment. Robert approved starting her on intravenous fluids to combat the dehydration and beginning a course of antibiotics to treat the likely infection, rationalizing that many older people can quickly become confused and lethargic with dehydration. Giving her fluids would test whether her condition was reversible, and if so, the antibiotics could help. We recognized that this was the first step down a slippery slope. Once treatment is begun, it is harder to stop it.

When there was no clinical response to the intravenous fluids and Ruth was unwilling to take anything by mouth, the nursing home staff suggested that we consider some type of feeding tube. This decision became the pivotal step. We agreed that we would draw our line in the sand at this point. While it might be reasonable to test the short-term benefits of fluids, there was no basis for attempting to sustain her life

artificially. As it happened, Ruth died before any further clinical actions were needed.

Although we had deviated somewhat from our plan for the end of
her life, we had remained in agreement. But our responses to her passing were very different. Robert was content to follow through with
the original plan for a memorial service later. For him, the death was
simply an incident. In effect, Ruth had died long before; if anything,
her death was a blessing for all concerned.

But Joan clearly needed closure right away. However much she
had anticipated and even rehearsed it, the actuality of Ruth's death
came as a great blow. Joan needed her family and friends around her.
Four of the five grandchildren and three of the great-grandchildren
gathered for a long weekend together days after Ruth's death. (Robert's
middle daughter, whose wedding Ruth had missed because of her
stroke, had had twins just a month earlier.) In addition, an outpour-
ing of friends and relatives attended a reception at Joan's house during
that weekend. Most of the grandchildren wanted to be there for their
own needs; they had their own grieving to do. Instead of the more formal memorial service we had imagined, her family gathered around
the kitchen table and talked about Ruth. It was an effective way of
obtaining closure and most participants seemed to feel better for the
experience.

The impromptu ceremony provided us with an opportunity to
recount anecdotes about Ruth and her family. The stories revealed
her to be a complex character, viewed quite differently by each of the
various narrators.

Most people remembered Ruth's glamour, as well as some of her
more difficult moments. She emerged as a colorful character, and her
humor was actively recalled. As the highlights of her life were remembered, one could almost imagine her asking who would play her in the

movie version of her life. One granddaughter talked about her love for her grandmother and how she felt especially close but realized that her grandmother's admiration of her was based in part on her looks. Both her son-in-law and her daughter-in-law recounted how Ruth had opposed their marriages to her children but both had become reconciled with her and felt strong bonds of affection. We also used the occasion to distribute some of her jewelry to her grandchildren and their spouses.

In a sense, writing this book together represents a way for us to put real closure on this history. Our mother would have been very pleased to know that her stroke and subsequent struggles resulted in a closeness and collaboration between us. She would have loved to be the subject of such a joint venture.

LESSONS

1   It is important to distinguish between advance directives and end-of-life decisions. The former may be made far in advance of impending death and are usually based on imagined situations. In contrast, end-of-life decisions occur much closer to the actual event, usually when the person is experiencing at least some of the consequences of the terminal state. Advance directives are useful to help medical personnel and family members manage the events at the end of an older person's life. It is helpful for family members to discuss specific values and preferences with older people in order to gain a clear understanding of what they want. But it is vital, also, to recognize that the values that under- lie an advance directive may change when the person actually confronts the reality. Family members who are helping an older person make advance directives should keep in mind that people

are much more adaptable than we believe possible, and that one should not sign away one's options too readily.

2   Research has shown that states that people believe would be un-endurable are in fact quite well tolerated. As Shakespeare notes in *Macbeth*, "Present fears are less than horrible imaginings."

3   It is, therefore, useful to distinguish between advance directives made while people are still well, and that may reflect their fears about becoming severely ill, and end-of-life decisions made closer to the time of their actual death, when they have a better grasp of the meaning of the choices they make. At the point when frail older people truly believe that their current state of living is not one they want to go to great lengths to preserve, they should be helped to make whatever advance directives they feel comfort-able making.

4   Discussions about end-of-life care may stir up some strong family controversies. These issues are better aired and discussed than left to smolder.

5   There are differences between observing the dying process close up and day-to-day and doing so long distance. hose who are removed may be able to resist giving care more than those who have to watch the person die.

6   It takes a much longer time to die than one might think. Once a decision has been made to stop treatment, death may not come quickly.

7   Having advance directives does not always mean following them. A family member who has been vested with durable power of attorney may discover that what has been decided in theory may be difficult to put into practice when the time comes. Taking action is much easier, however, when there is consensus among family members. Family members should discuss their thoughts about appropriate end-of-life behavior well before the time comes to act.

8   The actual period around an older person's dying can bring out latent problems in family dynamics. It is better to anticipate and resolve such conflicts before they cloud discussions around end-of-life actions.

9   Even with advance planning and discussion, managing this critical period is extremely taxing.

10   Funerals and other forms of memorial service, formal or informal, can play an important role. Some act of closure is needed even when the death is anticipated.

11   People react to a loss of loved ones differently. All reactions are legitimate, and each person's needs must be addressed appropriately.

12

What Kind of Long-Term Care
Do We Want?
What Can We Do About It?

The message of this sad tale is that for families caring for their elderly, money and knowledge are necessary but not sufficient. In many respects our mother had a better chance at success than most other people in her circumstances. She was not wealthy but she could afford to pay privately for her care, although her resources would not cover as much private-duty nursing as might have been required and could not have lasted indefinitely. We, her two children, were assertive and knowledgeable, and we shared common goals and philosophies about care.

Even with all these advantages, her story is not a happy one. What chance then does the average person have? While it is better to have money to pay for long-term care and to know what to ask from the system, those advantages will not ensure that families will get the kind of care they want. It is essential that every family member become an aggressive advocate for the elderly person in need of long-term care.

But fighting the battle one case at a time is not enough to fix the system. Bigger changes are needed. These changes will require collective action from those who have had to suffer through dealing with an ineffective care system, from those who operate such a system, and from those who make the rules about how to regulate and pay for such a system.

The individual lessons of each stage in the saga of our mother's last years need to be viewed in the light of what is happening to long-term care in general in this country. Long-term care is a tough marketplace for the ill-prepared buyer, and most consumers are neophytes. Even as the very sophisticated consumers we considered ourselves, it was hard to get the kind of care we wanted. Involvement and advocacy, even enlightened advocacy, is not enough. Clearly, the system is broken and needs to be fixed. It is not just a question of being able to buy more care and more caring. Americans are too quick to think that everything boils down to money. We are already paying much more for all sorts of care and getting less back in return than are other countries. It is time to look at the system to determine how we can get our money's worth.

What Kind of Long-Term Care Do We Want?

Long-term care today is a national embarrassment. Although at least half of the adults alive today will need some form of long-term care and almost all of us will experience it as family members, little has been done to change the fundamental elements of the system. It should not be necessary to have to choose between having a livable, personalized environment and getting personal care. The touchstone of long-term care is still the nursing home.

Growing frail, becoming disabled, and losing one's mind is not a happy prospect. No amount of care is likely to reverse this terrible process, but much can be done to mitigate the suffering associated with this deterioration. As a first principle, the care provided should be designed to improve, not aggravate, the situation. Providing such care requires a rare blend of compassion and competence. But despite its rarity, such care has not been well rewarded, at least for those on the front line. Many nursing-home owners and operators may have grown wealthy living off the misery of others but the dedicated care-givers who provide the basic services needed to maintain frail older persons have not been paid well; nor has their contribution been accorded much social respect. If things are going to improve, they will have to start there.

Long-term care in America was never planned. It just evolved. What began as a small personal business changed its nature when substantial external funding became available with the creation of Medicaid in 1965. The nursing home suddenly became a real entity. Much of our subsequent long-term care activity has been directed toward dealing with that reality.

The nursing home was never invented as such. Early models were, effectively, extended boarding houses. The entry of Medicaid changed all that. The framers of Medicaid never expected that the program would be a major vehicle to cover the cost of nursing homes. They envisioned it as primarily a program to address the needs of poor mothers and their children. They forgot somehow that the poorest sector of society in the mid 1960s was the frail elderly.

Caught unaware, they were unprepared. A federal program needed regulations, especially about safety. The most available model regulations that covered facilities of about the same size were the life-safety

codes for small rural hospitals. Not surprisingly, then, the first generation of nursing homes came to resemble small hospitals.

But nursing homes are not hospitals. The basic social contract is
quite different. People who enter a hospital agree (at least tacitly) to
temporarily give up their identity, their dignity, and their control over
their life, in exchange for a reasonable shot at getting better. They endure the indignity of wearing those horrible gowns, being awakened
at all hours, and sharing a room with a stranger because it is only for
short time and because it seems to be the price one has to pay to get
better.

If this deal with the hospital seems Faustian, the bargain with a
nursing home is worse. The stays are often life sentences. The likelihood of benefit is much less. Basically, the environment is the treatment. Not surprisingly, few people agree to go to a nursing home if
they think they have any choice in the matter. The nursing home is the
last refuge.

Likewise, for decades public policy has been directed toward
seeking alternatives to nursing home care, first in the community by
supporting home care and more recently through institutions that
provide some form of assisted living. When given the opportunity,
many older people and their families have chosen these alternatives.
Often, however, they have proven to be less alternatives than tempo-
rary stopgaps. The growth in home care did not lead to a reduction
in the use of nursing homes. In contrast, assisted living did appear to
divert potential nursing home clients. Indeed, this strong consumer
response made assisted living a growth industry.

This very pattern of success raised new problems. Assisted-
living facilities sprang up all over. Most were operated by organizations that had little or no experience in personal care. The emphasis

was more on providing hotel services than on providing care. Although the original concept of assisted living was intended to address the deficiencies of nursing home care, the worst of which was the lack of respect for the privacy and autonomy of the resident, each new wave of assisted living offered a new variant. It was not long before the name lost all meaning. Almost any form of housing with some service operated under that name.

To the extent that assisted living was attempted to serve a population comparable to those served by nursing homes, a policy dilemma arose. Should not this new form of care be held to the same standards as nursing homes, which were stringently regulated after a series of scandals that uncovered very deficient care? Assisted-living proponents argued that the regulations had helped to shape nursing homes into the impersonal institutions they were. Imposing the same regulations on assisted living would simply transform them into nursing homes. The nursing home industry complained that the playing field was not level. Why should they be held to a higher standard? Outside observers worried that an unregulated assisted-living industry would force us to relive the checkered past of nursing homes.

To some extent, the issue is moot at the moment because assisted living and nursing homes do not really serve the same range of clientele. Although there is some overlap and there are some exceptions, assisted living serves primarily a spectrum of less disabled clients than do nursing homes. Assisted living currently markets primarily to a group of older persons who are still quite autonomous but do not want the burden of running their own household. Rather than gradually expanding the extent of care to meet the changing needs of clients, most assisted-living facilities discharge residents once their care needs become heavy. Others encourage families to take on the additional care burden by hiring personal care workers to serve one client exclusively. In effect, they are recreating a home care program within their institution. However, this option is expensive and inefficient.

Whereas nursing homes are effectively the creation of Medicaid and receive a substantial proportion of their revenues from this welfare program, assisted living is still largely a privately funded enterprise. A growing number of states are beginning to cover some forms of assisted living but, especially in the light of clear definitions of who is served and what constitutes a service, most of the states that do cover assisted living under Medicaid do so modestly.

Perhaps we should look upon assisted living as more a goal than an actuality. In a country as rich as ours it should not be necessary to choose between humane, livable care and technically competent care. We can afford both and should demand it. The real question is why we have tolerated not having it for so long. Part of the answer may lie in our low expectations of long-term care. But times are changing.

As the number of frail older persons living in the United States grows, the pressure to find a humane and affordable way to care for them will mount. Most people want to stay in their own homes as long as they can. Some combination of home care and family care (euphemistically called informal care) may serve them. But at some point the care needs become great enough that extended care is required. Providing long periods of such care by a single individual is very expensive. Moreover, home care must always weigh the costs of travel against the costs of care. Especially when the costs of care are borne by the public, it makes sense that at some point receiving care necessitates moving into a congregate living situation, where care can be provided more efficiently. The challenge is to design such situations so that these care recipients do not have to surrender their rights as individuals to receive this care. A country as creative as ours should surely be able to design an affordable and effective way of delivering care that retains a person's sense of being a person.

Managing people with dementia, especially advanced dementia, represents a special challenge. Many efforts have been made to create special care units for demented persons within nursing homes. Some assisted-living facilities offer such units as well. The underlying concept is to create an environment and a staff that is specifically suited to these people. Unfortunately, most of the studies of these special care units have failed to show any benefit. Reminiscent of the way we have historically treated mental illness, the major benefit is that they remove these disruptive clients from the rest of the client population and thereby may improve the quality of life for the more cognitively intact.

Clustering demented people, however, may create an environment that offers new burdens to at least some of them, as it did to our mother, who hated the idea of living among "crazy people." Who knows how many of those in special dementia units feel the same way? Despite (perhaps because of) the catchy names (e.g., reminiscence unit) and a décor that suggests an intention to encourage these people to relate to events from their childhood, these places may serve simply to isolate these disruptive elements.

Despite all of our credentials and education, we found the system unfriendly and difficult to navigate. It simply could not deliver the combination of competence and compassion that we sought. It was neither flexible nor resilient. We were looking less for highly trained professionals than for people who could solve problems, staff who were willing to think about what underlay the immediate behaviors, were observant to minimal changes in behavior, and recognized those as cues that some type of intervention was needed before a crisis arose. Perhaps that level of insight does require education, but training alone will not produce it. It requires an environment that is less concerned about litigation and sanction and more focused on making life worth living.

It should be reasonable to expect that quality of care and quality of life can be offered simultaneously. Institutions should not demand the loss of one's personhood as the price of admission. Certainly it would be unrealistic to expect that all care can be individualized, at least not with finite resources. Nonetheless, much more can be done to provide care in a livable environment, one that preserves residents' dignity and tries to accommodate their preferences as much as possible.

We have not begun to tap the depths of creativity in thinking about how to delivery affordable, livable, high-quality long-term care. A promising step seems to be the increasing use of nurse practitioners, who can provide medical care that is more personal and continuous than the sporadic, crisis-driven contacts most of the frail elderly now receive from physicians. The care nurse practitioners provide needs to be augmented by systematic ways to monitor the clinical status of long-term-care users and to trigger rapid-response interventions *before* the crises occur.

Caring for our mother through all of her tempests and turmoil strained our patience and left us frustrated and exhausted. Ruth was a difficult person to deal with when she was whole; she was even more difficult when her illness overwhelmed her inhibitions. There are thousands of Ruths out there. The people, like us, who work diligently to try to make their lives better should be rewarded and encouraged, not dismissed.

Making long-term care decisions, many of which must be made under great time pressure, is hard. There is rarely a right or wrong answer. The best answer must take into account and try to balance safety, comfort, medical oversight, control, and autonomy. Rarely do individuals or families closely examine their priorities. Even less often do they discuss them. Having such discussions can open old wounds and raise long-buried issues.

Dealing with complex family dynamics and conflicting priorities is hard enough under the best of circumstances. It is virtually impossible under pressure. If families have to make a decision by the end of the day, it is unlikely they can explore all the available options, let alone their feelings.

Making good long-term care decisions requires information (about the likely outcomes of various alternatives), clarity about the outcomes that are being prioritized, and time. It also requires outside help. Few families can deal with all this on their own. They need structure and support. Books and the Internet can provide information but not emotional support or the needed structure for the complete decision-making process. Trained individuals who are familiar with long-term care and know how to structure the steps in decision-making can be invaluable at this stage. They can help families separate the issues around which type of care is most appropriate from the question of which specific agency or institution is best suited to provide that care. Indeed, different criteria apply at each stage in the process. The same counselors can also help families to access specific information about the alternative expected courses under different treatment scenarios and the attributes of the various care providers. Unfortunately, the current system makes no provision for either the infrastructure to help organize this painful and complex decision-making or the personnel trained to provide the needed assistance.

What Can We Do?

Good long-term care will cost money. Since it is hands-on care, it will require more and better trained hands. For example, a recent federal study suggests that substantially more staff are needed in nursing homes to make them even potentially able to improve care.* But this additional staff carries a price tag that the federal government was not willing to bear, and hence the recommendation was squelched. Long-term care is hard work. It is physically and emotionally taxing. It often requires dealing with some of the most personal aspects of life. Yet the key caregivers are paid a pittance. It will probably never be possible to raise wages and benefits to a level that will attract people into this field, but at least we should be sure that good people who do enter do not leave because they can make more money dishing out fast food.

Making long-term care a more satisfying career for the care-givers will require more than money to provide better pay. If long-term care is ever to achieve the lofty goals that we seek, it must first be seen by all, including those who work in it, as a noble calling. It cannot be viewed as staffed by the rejects of other enterprises. The people who come to long-term care are frail and at the end of life's course. No amount of care can reverse much of that inevitability. While one can hope to maximize the quality of their lives and perhaps to even delay the rate at which their physical function deteriorates, the struggle is uphill. The measure of long-term care lies in its ability to slow decline and to preserve a sense that life still has value to the individual living it.

The triumph implied, however, by reducing the rate of decline.

---

*Abt Associates, Inc., Appropriateness of minimum nurse staffing ratios in nursing homes: Report to Congress—Phase II final report (Cambridge, MA: Abt Associates, Inc., 2001).

Such a triumph goes unnoticed unless special efforts are made to detect it. Because the overall outcome is still one of continual decline, recognizing this achievement means being able to compare what would have happened in the absence of good care to what did happen. This difference is much harder to demonstrate than showing how good care saved a life. It requires having good data on what happens to most frail people as they decline against which to contrast the effects of good care.

Although good investment in long-term care can often bring about greater dividends than a comparable investment in futile acute care, those who provide long-term care are generally rewarded and recognized dramatically less than those who provide acute care. Unless we plan to start looking for large ice floes on which to launch our growing frail older population, we had best begin to think of ways to make long-term care a more rewarding and respected career. Someday our lives may depend on that step.

People with private funds will probably always get more than those who rely on government programs, but we should establish a floor of care that is available to everyone who needs it. Our story demonstrates that having resources does not guarantee good (even reasonable) care.

Getting a better long-term care system means becoming better individual customers and developing a stronger collective consumer presence overall. Individual consumerism is necessary but not sufficient. Too many forces shape the current system to allow it to adapt as it should. Unfortunately long-term care is an area where most people have little practice or experience. The various how-to books that are written to help families cope offer some practical advice but they are usually quite detached from the emotional realities of the experience. (See Appendix 1.) We have tried to provide some basic lessons from our experience but these are more often cautions than solutions. The problems will not get easier until the care gets better.

Long-term care needs to be on the political agenda. Today no politician seems willing to tackle this issue or even to acknowledge it. Nor are politicians ever likely to take up this banner unless they are pressed to do so by a vitalized constituency. We need to create a mood of creative intolerance, one that insists that the current situation will not suffice and demands that improvements are needed now.

Making change involves taking some risks. We have evolved a complex, burdensome set of regulations designed initially to protect and promote good care, but they have gotten out of hand. We need to roll them back and shift attention from prescribing every action and the qualifications for every actor to holding the system accountable at a higher level of abstraction for achieving reasonable outcomes. These outcomes include both quality of life and quality of care. It is unrealistic to seek zero-fault programs. We should be comfortable with lowering the rate of bad events and rewarding the occurrence of good ones. We will never reward what we cannot measure. We need to employ the measures of quality of life with the same vigor we now apply to quality-of-care measures.

No organized voice speaks for long-term care consumers and their families. Most nonprofit advocacy groups are organized around a specific disease. Some, like the Alzheimer's Association, recognize the centrality of long-term care but their agenda is focused on finding a cure or a better treatment for the disease. The American Association of Retired Persons has become more vocal about long-term care but has given much more attention to prescription drug coverage.

The time has come to create a national organization to build a groundswell of concern and attention for long-term care. Such a group could be modeled on the Alzheimer's Association, which draws its strength from a partnership of lay people (largely family members of current or deceased victims) and health and social service professionals who are dedicated to improving care. These same components are available for long-term care in even greater numbers.

This new National Association to Improve Long-term Care should begin by making long-term care a central issue. It can work to inform the general public about the current problems and the evidence that good care can make a big difference. It should lobby Congress to insist on better care, including a will to pay for it. It should provide families who must deal with this crisis a place to come for practical information as well as support. Among its planks should be the following:

- Good long-term care makes a big differences in the lives of those who need it and their families.
- It should not be necessary to trade quality of life against quality of care.
- To encourage broader coverage, separate payment for services provided from that for room and board. In essence, a person could live in various congregate settings and receive the same level and types of supportive services.
- Most people want to stay in their homes as long as possible, but at some point efficiency will mandate that they move into some form of congregate care.
- Good care does not happen by accident. It must be actively pursued.
- Regulations are undoubtedly necessary to provide sufficient safeguards but they must not interfere with innovation and aiming high. Floors too readily become ceilings.

- Most people who need long-term care have complex medical problems. Good long-term care must interface effectively with medical care.
- Good care should be rewarded. Those organizations that can show they make a difference in people's lives should be acknowledged and perhaps paid more.
- Universal long-term care is feasible. Other countries have developed universal programs that cover long-term care. Some use public monies; others use a combination of public and private money.

Those who provide care need to be permitted, and even encouraged, to take a new look at what they do. Much of what has become the lore of long-term care needs to be challenged. Just because things have been done a certain way does not make that way best. Good providers need to be given the tools to provide better care. Systems that allow people to take risks without putting them at jeopardy need to be created. The concept of managed risk, which implies accepting some potential consequences of decisions that call for less care or more autonomy, has a real role to play. Many advocates fear that allowing such risks is the first step to perdition. Alternatively, many providers now see themselves faced with real risks of bankrupting litigation if they stray from the path of orthodoxy.

All of us who have been through the long-term care experience can testify to the failings of the current system. It is time we did something to make sure that when we become the generation in need of long-term care neither we nor our children will have to contend with these failings.

Appendix 1
Suggested Reading

Adamec, Chris. *The Unofficial Guide to Eldercare*. New York: Macmillan, 1999.
> This broad how-to book, written by a journalist, provides basic information that can help with decision making. It includes long-term care (nursing home and assisted living) and refers to specific studies.

Beerman , Susan, and Judith Rappaport-Musson. *Eldercare 911*. Amherst, NY: Proetheus, 2002.
> This book was written by professionals to provide caregivers with practical tips, simple worksheets, and guides.

Cohen, Donna, and Carl Eisdorfer. *Caring for Your Aging Parents*. New York: Tarcher Putnam, 1993.
> Written by two gerontologists, this book offers general advice on caregiving and seven steps to effective parent care.

Ilardo, Joseph, and Carole Rothman. *Are Your Parents Driving You Crazy?* Acton, MA: Vander Wyk & Burnham, 2001.
> This book is written by professionals to help readers deal with specific dilemmas.

Lebow, Grace, Irwin Lebow, and Barbara Kane. *Coping with Your Difficult Older Parent*. New York: Avon Books, 1999.
> Written by a trio of professionals (none related to us), this book provides general strategies for dealing with difficult situations but does not specifically address long-term care.

Lieberman, Trudy and the editors of *Consumer Reports*. *Complete Guide to Health Services for Seniors*. New York: Three Rivers Press, 2000.
> This comprehensive and practical volume addresses several salient issues, including paying for health care, finding long-term care, and paying for long-term care. It provides worksheets and reference material.

Loverde, Joy. *Complete Eldercare Planner*. 2nd ed. New York: Hyperion, 1997.
> Written by a journalist, this book offers broad advice across a wide spectrum of issues. Its coverage of long-term care is less complete.

Markut, Lynda A., and Anatole Crane. *Dementia Caregivers Share Their Stories: A Support Book in a Book*. Nashville: Vanderbilt University Press, 2005.
> This book is filled with inspirational stories, practical advice, and creative approaches to the challenges of caregiving.

Morris, Virginia. *How to Care for Your Aging Parents*. New York: Workman, 1996.
> Written by a journalist, this how-to book covers a wide range of issues. It has a useful section on choosing a nursing home but is less good on assisted living. It is not as thorough as Adamec, *Unofficial Guide*.

Rhodes, Linda Colvin. *Complete Idiot's Guide: Caring for Aging Parents*. Indianapolis: Alpha Books, 2000.
> Written by a professional, this book offers basic information, along with strategies and tips.

Appendix 2
Web-Based Resources on Long-Term Care

AARP [American Association of Retired Persons] National Organization

www.aarp.org

> Provides information on AARP member benefits, legislative issues, and life transitions.

Administration on Aging

www.aoa.gov

> The Administration on Aging Web site provides specific ways to contact more local resources such as on state units on aging and area agencies on aging.

Alzheimer's Association

www.alz.org

> *Residential Care: A Guide for Choosing a New Home* is published by the Alzheimer's Association for families looking for residential care for someone with Alzheimer's Disease. Call 1-800-272-3900 for a free copy.

American Association of Homes and Services for the Aging (AAHSA)

www.aahsa.org/public/consumer.htm

> AAHSA is a national organization consisting of more than five thousand not-for-profit nursing homes, continuing care retirement communities, senior housing and assisted living facilities, and community services. This site provides tips on choosing facilities and services as well as a searchable directory.

American Health Care Association (AHCA)
www.ahca.org

> AHCA is a nonprofit federation of affiliated state health organizations, together representing nearly twelve thousand nonprofit and for-profit assisted living, nursing facility, developmentally disabled, and subacute care providers that care for more than 1.5 million elderly and disabled individuals nationally.

CareGuide
www.eldercare.com

> Features a full range of services, articles, and resources for elder care. Visitors can explore the site via the Resource Guide, or find content by taking an elder situation assessment.

CarePlanner
www.careplanner.org

> A decision-support tool for successful living and care choices for seniors, caregivers, family, friends, and professionals.

Centers for Medicare and Medicaid Services (CMS)
www.medicare.gov/nhcompare/home.asp

> CMS (formerly the Health Care Financing Administration) is the federal agency that oversees Medicare and Medicaid. This site is the homepage for Nursing Home Compare; it provides rudimentary information about all Medicare and Medicaid nursing homes by city and state and how they performed on their last inspection; a directory of state long-term care ombudsman programs and state survey agencies, and other useful information. It includes A Guide to Choosing a Nursing Home.

Eldercare Locator
www.eldercare.gov

> Nationwide directory of state and local area agencies on aging and community-based organizations that can direct older adults and their caregivers to sources of care.

National Association of Home Care
www.nahc.org

> Contains information relevant to the interests of the home care and

hospice community and tips for consumers on choosing a home care provider.

National Center for Assisted Living (NCAL)
www.ncal.org
NCAL is the assisted living voice of the American Health Care Association, the nation's largest organization representing long-term care. The Web site provides general advice about assisted living.

National Citizens' Coalition for Nursing Home Reform
www.nccnhr.org/
Their *Consumer Guide to Choosing a Nursing Home* includes a checklist for selecting a nursing home and other information for families who want quality nursing home care. This and other publications are available from the National Citizens' Coalition for Nursing Home Reform.

National Council on the Aging
www.ncoa.org
The National Council on Aging is a complex organization that addresses many issues related to aging, depression, employment, family care, health care, hearing impairment, housing, long-term care, pain, personal finance, religion and spirituality, substance abuse, and sexuality. The Web site provides general advice on a variety of topics.

National Long Term Care Ombudsman Resource Center
www.ltcombudsman.org
Provides information about a national team of volunteers who visit residents of long-term care facilities to offer friendship and to listen to concerns and problems; provides a link for locating local ombudsmen.

Senior Law
www.seniorlaw.com
Provides access to information about elder law, Medicare, Medicaid, estate planning, trusts, and the rights of the elderly and disabled.

Index